THE TRUTH ABOUT CORE TRAINING

Discover the dark side of conventional abdominal exercises and
train your core smarter with the Hypopressive Method

Illustrations: Levent Efe
Book and cover design: www.watersdesigns.com.au

Paperback: 978-0-6459171-0-9
eBook: 978-0-6459171-1-6

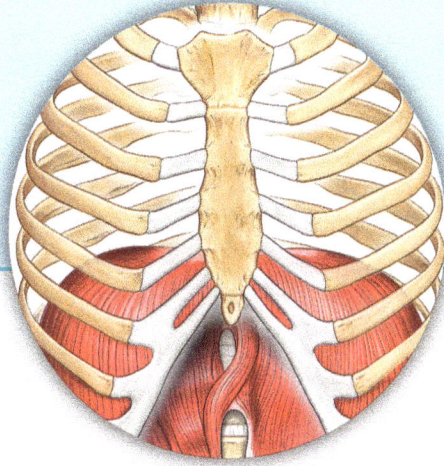

THE TRUTH ABOUT CORE TRAINING

Discover the dark side of conventional abdominal exercises and train your core smarter with the Hypopressive Method

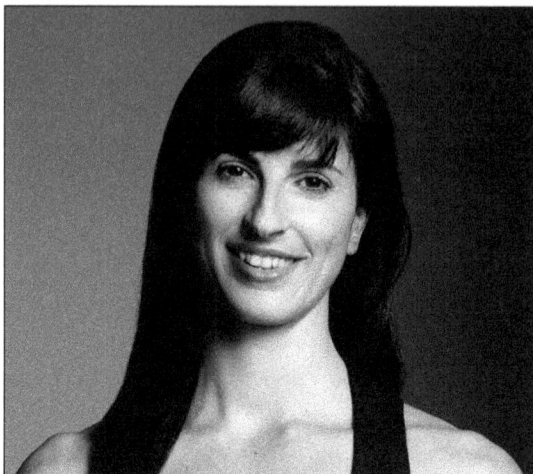

Paula was born and raised in Spain, where she became a professional Pole Vaulter while completing her Bachelor in Sports Science and Masters in Sports Performance. Through her studies, Paula discovered the Hypopressive Method, a new technique revolutionising core training and pelvic floor function.

In 2012, Paula moved to Australia and started her journey in the fitness industry, first as a Pilates Instructor and then as a studio owner. This progression allowed Paula to introduce Hypopressive Training to both clients and other fitness and health professionals interested in improving their clients' quality of life.

As a mother of two, Paula's passion is to educate women in core and pelvic health to prevent the most common conditions related to pregnancy, post-partum and menopause.

To Mum,
wherever you are in the universe.

To my two miracles,
Lola and Paco.

ACKNOWLEDGEMENTS:

Thank you to everyone who has been directly and indirectly involved
in the creation of this book, from those who guided me in this adventure
to those who looked after my young children so I could have some time
to make this project a reality.

Mike, your belief in me and the seed you planted in my head
have been instrumental in this journey.
Thank you.

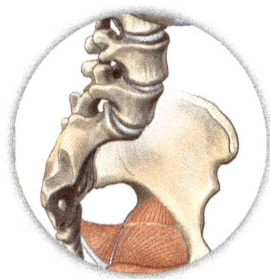

THE TRUTH ABOUT CORE TRAINING

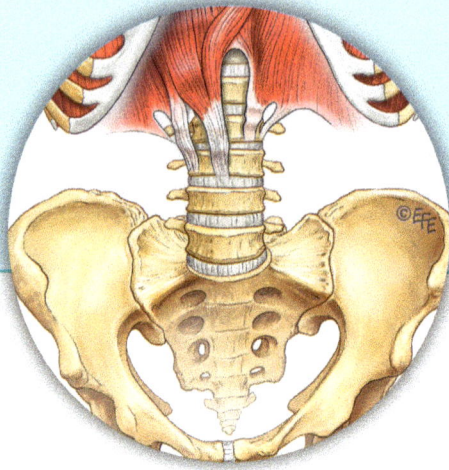

THE TRUTH
ABOUT CORE TRAINING

IN

THE TRUTH ABOUT CORE TRAINING
WHY IS IT **IMPORTANT** TO TRAIN YOUR CORE?

It goes without saying that individuals neglect what they take for granted, which applies to everything from relationships to work to healthy bodily functions. In many cases, some people's cars are better maintained than their bodies.

But there is one problem that affects virtually everyone – gravity. Yes, gravity! That unending force which constantly works against our spine, posture and core, and yet also encourages our digestive system to flow downhill. When we breathe, eat and drink, an entire group of muscles come into play, some of which continue to operate afterwards. All major operating parts – digestion, reproduction and urination – are located in the abdominal cavity in what we commonly refer to as the core.

GRAVITY works against the muscles of the core, and with the addition of pregnancy, unwanted weight, or a sedentary lifestyle, the core muscles begin to malfunction if we do not take proper care of them.

Ironically, a visit to the gym isn't always the solution, especially if we don't know what we are doing. You would be surprised by the number of people suffering from the consequences of dysfunctional core muscles due to incorrect training strategies.

There is a strong relationship between how fit your core is and whether you suffer from STRESS URINARY INCONTINENCE or have a weak pelvic floor.

THE STATS:

- Stress Urinary Incontinence (SUI) is reported to affect around 16–21% of women in Australia. With most being middle aged (34–44 years). That is roughly 2.3 million women.[1]

- The rates of women seeking help are low; only 25% of women with incontinence have sought help for their symptoms.[2]

- Pelvic Organ Prolapse (POP) is prevalent in up to 50% of women over forty and up to 75% of women attending gynaecology clinics.[3] POP is a major health issue that significantly impacts the quality of life for women. Surgery is currently the go-to treatment for POP but it is not always successful. There is a clear necessity for effective, low-risk and low-cost treatment strategies for POP.

- Female athletes and other physically active individuals are likely to experience stress urinary incontinence.[4]

- There is a significant association between low back pain and stress urinary incontinence.[5]

As a former professional pole vaulter, I suffered the consequences of thirteen years of high-impact activities and heavy weightlifting before learning how to train my core effectively. I was stronger than most of my male friends and was the envy of my brother for my extremely well-defined "six pack" and biceps, but my body was showing signs of internal weakness without me realising it. Whenever my training involved any sort of intense jumping, I would pack a spare pair of underwear and tights so I could continue my training session without being embarrassed by a tell-tale wet patch. I was in my early twenties.

One female in my training group had enough courage to eventually inform our male coach that the jumps were causing her to wet herself involuntarily. It goes without saying that our male training mates roared with laughter, believing it was because she was the oldest member of the training group. I decided to remain quiet and deal with my problem in silence, though I was relieved I wasn't the only one dealing with it. In retrospect, I now realise that I had been suffering from stress urinary incontinence since the age of 15. I had never thought it was an issue because my mom had the same problem, and she said it was normal. I didn't worry about it, let alone ask for help or advice. And here lies a large part of the problem. Most women consider it quite normal to leak urine when coughing, sneezing or exercising, have a pelvic organ prolapse after childbirth, or have a back or abdominal hernia.

ALL THESE DISORDERS ARE COMMON, BUT NOT THE NORMAL, HEALTHY WAY A BODY FUNCTIONS.

The fact that pelvic floor disorders are common does not make them okay, and it does not mean that we don't need to find a way to solve them. With my University Degrees in Physical Activity, Health and Sports Performance, I believed I had a good understanding of the human body and its functions. However, I wasn't even aware I had minimal understanding of pelvic health.

The topic is so obscure that even female instructors, coaches and therapists are unaware of the special care this area needs, for both men and women. Most fitness and sports qualifications do not provide enough education about core and pelvic health, yet a high proportion of our athletes and clients suffer from some sort of dysfunction in the area. Worse, because low back pain is often due to a weak pelvic floor, when coaches and trainers prescribe "abdominal" exercises to support the back, they can unknowingly aggravate the underlying issue, and potentially make it worse.

Furthermore, nowadays most believe in the equality of sexes and extrapolate that to mean women and men can train and do the same exercises, which is true to a point. But we have to recognise that we have some anatomical differences that must be considered so women can train using the same strategies as men and avoid injury. Fitness and health professionals need to stay on top of new research and information, always seeking greater insight and methods to support their clients. However, current motivation is usually driven by the individual's curiosity and motivation to provide the best they can for their clients and make a difference in their health. Hence, curiosity about pelvic and core health is usually triggered only when either the professionals or someone close to them experiences a core dysfunction or chronic pain after having a child.

This wasn't my case. After a knee injury ended my athletic career, I became interested in more sustainable forms of training and exercise. Based on my own experience, I concluded that if a training program leads to injury or stops you from exercising for several days because it is causing you pain, then it is unsustainable. (This does not include the mild, delayed muscle soreness that you can experience after a strength session).

My philosophy is that everybody needs to find a SUITABLE ACTIVITY for their individual fitness level that allows them to keep active for life.

During my years working in the fitness industry, I have come across many types of musculoskeletal dysfunctions and injuries. This has pushed me to learn more and more so I can help my clients achieve their fitness and health goals. Some issues were easier than others to manage, and my clients and I often worked with other health professionals to help them navigate and fix their issues. However, I always felt I was missing something when it came to core training. I felt like I didn't have enough information and couldn't answer the following questions:

- Why did many of my clients still complain about not having a flat stomach, even after doing two to three core training sessions a week and having a healthy diet and an active lifestyle?

- As a rule of thumb, all fitness professionals are told not to prescribe pregnant clients any crunch-based exercises or planks. What alternative did I have to train their core safely?

- If my clients supposedly have a strong core, why do they still complain of back pain?

In 2010, I took my father, who was recovering from prostate surgery, to visit an Osteopath, and the experience made me think more seriously about these questions.

My father was 58 years old and had previously undergone surgery for a herniated disc. Despite obviously never being pregnant, his overly large stomach had caused abdominal wall separation (known as abdominal diastasis) – more on this later.

My father had been regularly visiting this Osteopath to manage his back pain, and at the end of this session the Osteopath called me in to have a chat about Dad's training. To my surprise, he told me to eliminate any conventional core training from Dad's program. He explained that my father's abdominal wall could not handle this sort of movement and that his core training was possibly aggravating his abdominal diastasis. His pelvic floor and back muscles were simply too weak. Dumbfounded, I asked the Osteopath how I was meant to train my dad's core without using conventional core training techniques.

HIS ANSWER INTRODUCED ME TO A WHOLE NEW WORLD OF CORE TRAINING, IN PARTICULAR, THE TECHNIQUE KNOWN AS HYPOPRESSIVE TRAINING.

This technique was originally designed by Dr Marcel Caufriez to help women with incontinence, but people like my dad – and anyone with weak pelvic floor and core or back muscles – could benefit from its practice.

It is a holistic approach to core training based on postural function, core muscle synergy and its connection with one's breathing patterns.

The Osteopath taught me a couple of exercises to introduce into my dad's training program as a replacement for his conventional core training. After a couple of months, my father improved significantly, and started to feel much better without the traditional core training exercises. (The Hypopressive Techniques are in Chapter 11).

My Dad's experience led me to question whether we are doing the right thing with current training strategies. Do we really need to perform endless crunches to have a functional core? Is there any point in being able to hold a plank for minutes if we don't perform planks in our daily activities?

The different systems of our bodies – digestive, respiratory, reproductive, etc – are studied as if they are independent of each other, but the body works as a whole. Our organs, muscles, fascia, bones, and even our emotions, are all linked. The way we stand and breathe and how our muscles work in synergy when we move are very important. The abdominal wall, pelvic floor and breathing muscles do not work independently, so why do we train them separately?

I became more and more curious about hypopressive training and started a journey that commenced in Spain, learning all about the method from the first disciples of Marcel Caufriez and completing my qualifications to become a Hypopressives Master Trainer. I am now the founder of HYPOPRESSIVES AUSTRALIA, the only organisation in the country that teaches other fitness and health professionals this innovative method to improve the health and well-being of their clients.

This book is the result of many years of looking after not only my clients', but my own health. I have constantly learned and studied, searching for a better understanding of the human body, so I can find solutions to any disorders. I hope this book answers your questions about dysfunctions you may be dealing with and how core training can help. It is never too late to make changes to your health.

If you are a woman reading this book, please encourage the men in your life to read it too, because men also suffer the consequences of damaging core training choices. They can benefit from reading this book, not only for their own health, but also to gain greater insight into the issues that affect the women around them.

If you are a professional in the health and fitness area,

I invite you to read this book with an open mind.

Although some contents can be too basic for your level of knowledge,

you may find some valuable information in the different chapters

and the research attached.

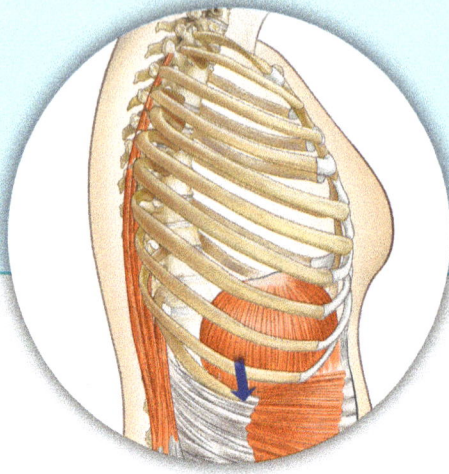

CHAPTER 01

BUSTING THE MYTH
OF CONVENTIAL CORE TRAINING

BUSTING THE MYTH OF CONVENTIONAL CORE TRAINING

01

CORE TRAINING IS **MORE** THAN COUNTING THE NUMBER OF CRUNCHES YOU DO EVERY DAY

Over the course of the history, scientific knowledge has evolved in response to questions, and solved many of the problems humanity faces. Health is one of the fields where science has evolved the most, as evidenced by the dramatic increase of life expectancy we've had over the past century. Thanks to vaccines and drugs, we can now cure and prevent many diseases that used to kill people, have greater access to health information and are more aware of the factors that create good health than ever before.

Nonetheless, in retrospect we are still sometimes surprised at the things we used to do because we thought they were good for us, but now know they aren't.

For example, health authorities used to advise us that eating excess fat was the reason for obesity and that we needed to consume low fat products or eliminate fat altogether. Now we know that refined sugars have a major impact on obesity and that not all fat is bad for us. In fact, now we know that to achieve a healthy weight we need to consider much more than just the amount of fat in our diets.

When it comes to pelvic floor and core training, we seem to be reproducing the training programs developed in the last century. Arnold Kegel first invented his "Kegel" exercises in 1948, which are a series of muscle clenching movements designed to strengthen the pelvic floor muscles. While clenching the pelvic floor every day does strengthen your pelvic floor, it doesn't really target anything else around and connected to it. The same happens when we think the only way to have a strong core is by performing endless abdominal crunch variations and planks. Especially when there are studies suggesting that curl-up movements can potentially aggravate pelvic floor disorders.[6] As with our diet, there are more aspects to be considered in core and pelvic floor training and a holistic and functional approach gives us better results than training them individually.

THERE IS A PRESSING NEED FOR CHANGE IN THE FITNESS AND HEALTH INDUSTRY AND IT IS TIME TO UPDATE SOME OF THE CONCEPTS ABOUT CORE TRAINING AND PELVIC FLOOR HEALTH.

WHAT DOES OUR CORE NEED TO BE ABLE TO DO?

Let's be realistic, your core isn't designed to perform endless crunches or planks. Think about how many minutes a day during your normal activities, you spend in a plank position or doing crunches. Probably not even a minute. We don't need to train our cores for that.

But what do you think your core is doing when you sit in front of your computer for eight hours a day, or when vacuuming your house or standing in the kitchen cooking dinner? It's providing stability. Therefore, TRAIN YOUR CORE FOR YOUR NEEDS.

One of the main principles of athletics training is the principle of "specificity or similarity", which means the training activities should be relevant to the discipline performed and the training movements should be similar to the movement performed in competition.

Simply explained, if you're a swimmer you need to swim to improve your performance, if you're a cyclist, you need to cycle. You wouldn't expect to become a good swimmer by riding a bicycle!

Think of yourself as an athlete who needs the best performance for your daily tasks. For example, if you spend most of your time sitting on a chair, you need to train your body to perform its best at sitting so you don't suffer from chronic back pain or other work-related injuries. If your job involves lifting heavy weights your core needs to be trained to provide support and the ability to modulate the tensions produced in your body when lifting the weights. When I had my first child, the tasks I needed my core to perform changed to being able to vacuum the house with my right hand while holding my clingy baby in my left arm, and not hurting my back while doing it.

WHAT IS THE CORE?

It's important to know what muscles make up the core before we go any further. In my first session with clients, I often ask them what they think the core is, and most of the time they hesitantly point to their bellies. I wish it was that simple, but there's a lot more happening in the centre of your body and there are many more muscles hiding behind that reflection in the mirror.

According to the Cambridge Dictionary, the word "core" means the basic and most important part of something. But it can also refer to the hard, central part of something, normally a fruit.

When referring to human anatomy, the Cambridge Dictionary defines the core as "the muscles around your pelvis, hips and abdomen that you use in most body movements".

With this simple definition we can already guess that the core consists of a much larger group of structures than the "6 pack". But you don't need to have an in-depth knowledge of your anatomy and physiology to have an informed understanding of what makes up the core and their functions.

Think of your core as a cylindrical structure. The front is your abdominal wall, the sides are your oblique muscles, you have the deep spinal muscles at the back and top, in the middle is the diaphragm (which is the main muscle we use for breathing) and at the base is your pelvic floor (the floor of your core).

Diaphragm

Transversus
abdominis m.

Erector
spinae
m.

Pelvic
floor

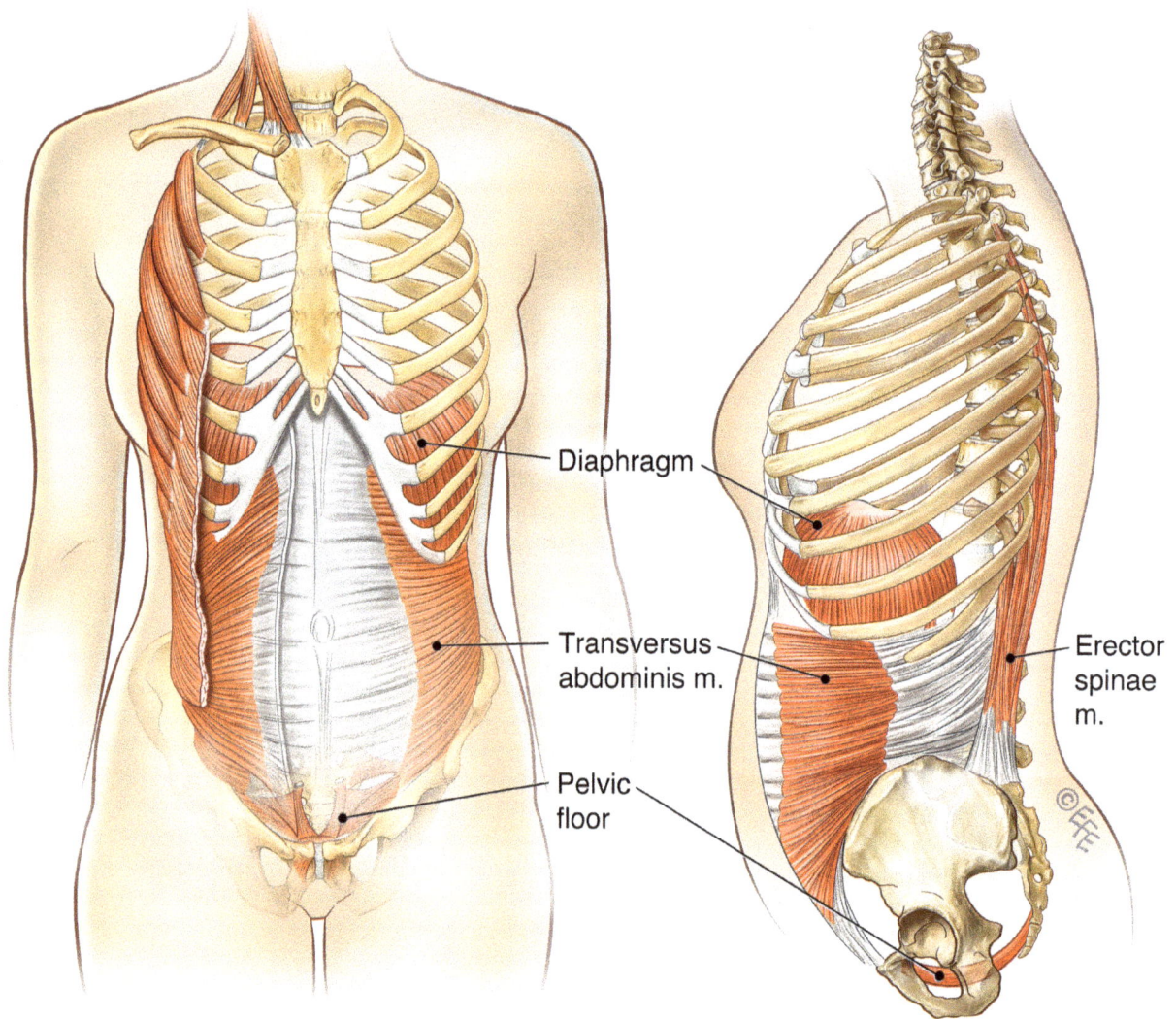

There is a muscle on your abdominal wall that requires special attention. It is called the **Transverus Abdominis.** As you can see, it is like a
wide belt that wraps around your waist acting as a corset.

It is also the deepest muscle in your abdominal wall and the main
muscle that participates in trunk stabilisation. Stability is one of its
functions, but this muscle also modulates the pressures produced in
your abdominal cavity when breathing, talking, coughing, moving, etc.

All parts of your core work in coordination to maintain the following functions:

- Stability in your body while static or moving

- Support of the internal organs in your abdominal and pelvic cavity

- Assistance with breathing patterns

You may have never thought about it, but inside your core —in your abdominal and pelvic cavities— is where some of the most important functions of your body occur.

They are:

- Breathing and phonation

- Digestion

- Sex and reproduction

- Continence

- Support

- Movement

- Blood circulation

THE GREAT MISCONCEPTION ABOUT CORE STABILITY[7]

The concept of core stability has become very popular over recent years. If you have ever experienced back pain, you have likely been told that you need to improve your core stability and have probably been prescribed a specific exercise program to reach this goal. This concept is often misunderstood and mismanaged.

Core stability refers to the core's natural ability to provide support to the entire body. Research has shown that trunk control has relevance in back pain and injury. However, this has led to a misconception that trunk bracing (tightening the muscles of the abdominal wall) is the key to preventing and even curing back pain and that a strong core will prevent injury. This isn't the case.

The constant bracing of the trunk leads to an abnormal state of continual contraction of your abdominal muscles that can cause the onset of other dysfunctions and pains and increase the compression of the lumbar spine. Holding your belly in restricts blood flow and can even interfere with digestion, bowel movement and the correct positioning of your abdominal and pelvic organs.

A study of pregnant women has shown no correlation between the ability to perform a sit-up and backache, which means that the strength of the abdominal muscle is not related to back pain. If it were true that only a strong "braced" core prevented back pain, then why is it that, despite experiencing the weight of the baby, the distension and the concomitant stretching of the abdominal muscles and tissues, do pregnant women not necessarily experience back pain?

> **WE CANNOT ASSUME THAT A STRONG CORE WILL AUTOMATICALLY FREE US FROM BACK PAIN.**

According to this belief, all overweight people should also have back pain, yet epidemiological studies have shown a weak link between these two factors.[8] Besides, skinny people have back pain too!

Having a strong core is important, but it's not only about core strength; we have overestimated the importance of the core for body stability. When you stand or walk, the muscles of your abdominal wall do not need to activate, on average, more than 5% of their maximum voluntary contraction.[9]

Furthermore, some studies have shown that during "core stability" exercises, the muscles don't activate at the intensity level needed to cause hypertrophy (muscle growth) and strength gain.[10,11]

The core muscles do not work independently of other trunk muscles and the other structures of the body, such as the fascia, bones, organs and nerves. Even when you move your arms, your core muscles respond, so how fast they "switch on" in response to the arm movement is vital (this term is called "timing").

The different structures of our bodies all need to work in synergy to provide appropriate anatomical and biomechanical support. Trying to isolate the core muscles from the rest of the body only leads to dysfunctional movement patterns and is likely to result in pain or injury.

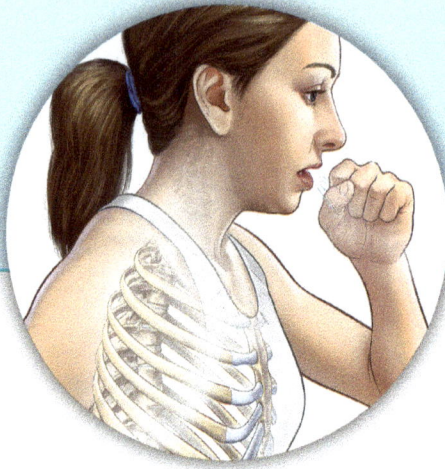

THE TWO KEY CONCEPTS OF SMART CORE TRAINING

02

THE TWO KEY CONCEPTS OF SMART CORE TRAINING

THERE IS AN **EXPLANATION** AS TO WHY YOU STILL NEED TO PULL YOUR BELLY IN TO KEEP YOUR BELLY FLAT DESPITE DOING ENDLESS CRUNCHES AT THE GYM

Two important factors in healthy core function are often overlooked but are crucial for our core's integrity and optimal performance. One is intra-abdominal pressure (IAP), and the other is muscle tone.

WHAT IS INTRA-ABDOMINAL PRESSURE?

You have probably never heard this term before, but it is present in every single activity of your daily life. And it plays an essential role in your core and pelvic floor function.

TO EXPERIENCE WHAT IAP IS, TRY THIS SIMPLE ACTION:

Close your hand into a fist and blow through it, noticing what happens to your belly and pelvic floor. Do you feel the pressure increasing in your stomach?

IAP increases every time you sneeze, cough, lift your baby, carry your groceries, run to catch the bus, lift weights, and even when talking or singing. The intra-abdominal pressure varies depending on the level of effort the task demands. How your core structures manage that pressure is vital for your core, pelvic and back health.

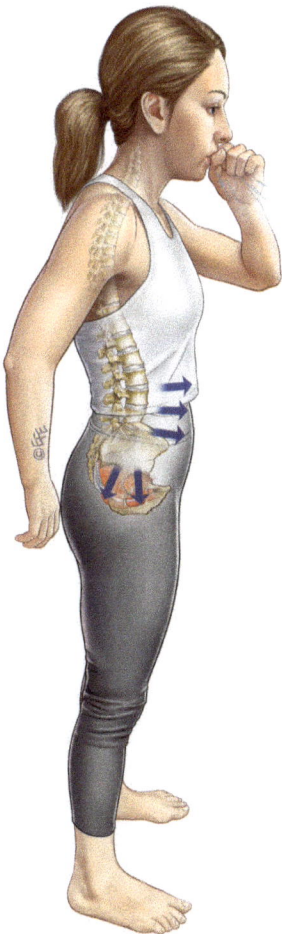

SO HOW DOES YOUR CORE RESPOND WHEN IAP INCREASES?

Imagine your abdominal cavity is a balloon. In a functional core, when the pressure increases, for example when you cough, the pressure generated in your abdominal cavity will push towards the sacrum, the coccix and the posterior muscles of the pelvic floor (levator ani muscles). These structures are strong enough to withstand the increase of pressure.

But what happens when the core is not functional? The pressure changes its direction and instead of pushing towards the back of the pelvic cavity will do it towards the front, which has smaller and weaker muscles that are not designed to withstand such amount of pressure.

Body alignment and posture plays an important role on the distribution of the intra abdominal pressure at rest and during a movement. We will talk more in depth about this later in the book.

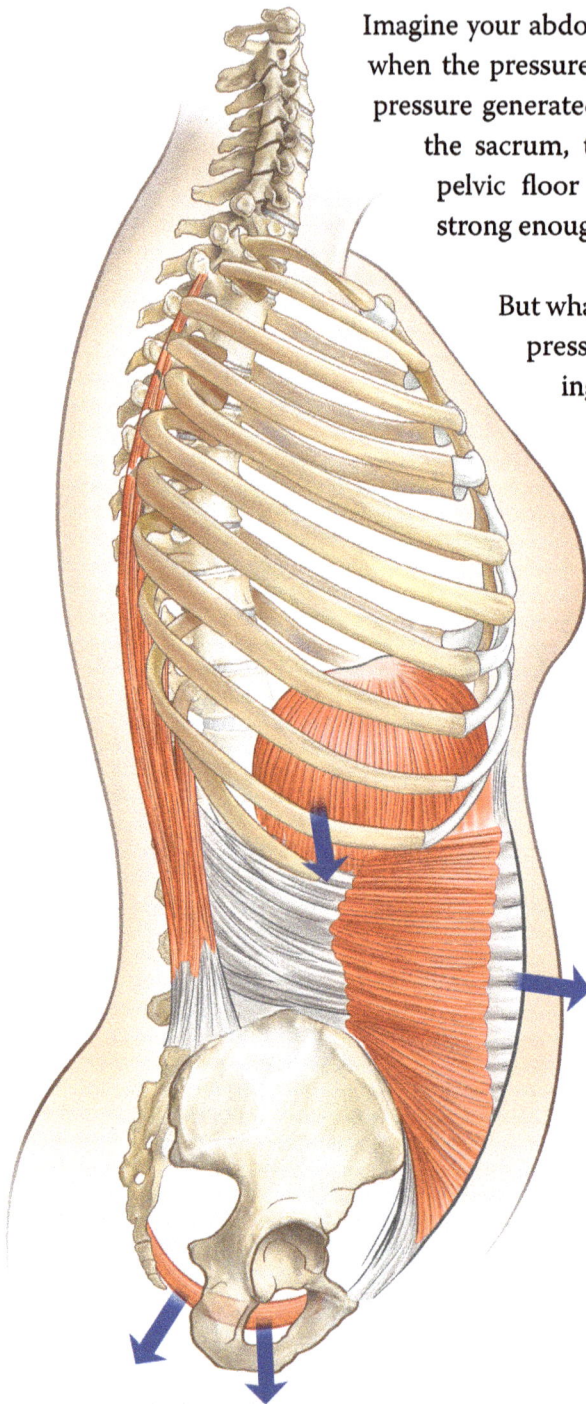

A SIMPLE WAY TO FIND OUT IF YOUR CORE AND PELVIC FLOOR ARE FUNCTIONING CORRECTLY IS BY DOING THE "COUGH TEST".

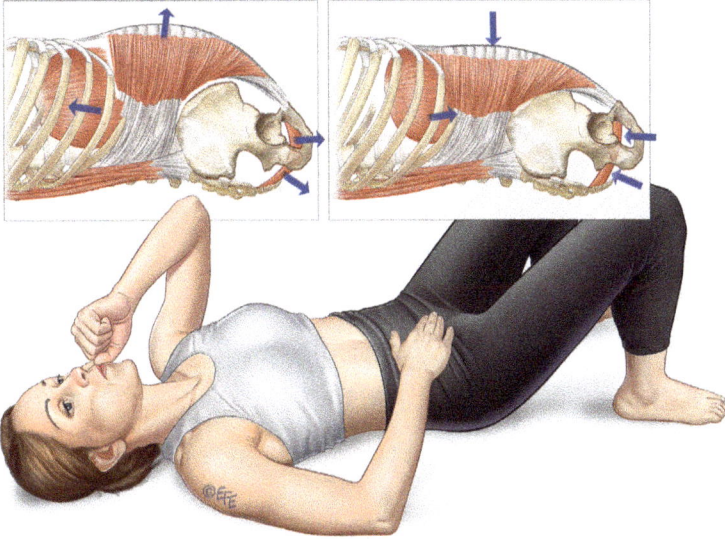

Test One

Lie on your back and place your hand between your belly button and pubic bone. Cough and notice the movement your stomach makes. Did it push your hand up, did your hand stay still, or did it draw it down?

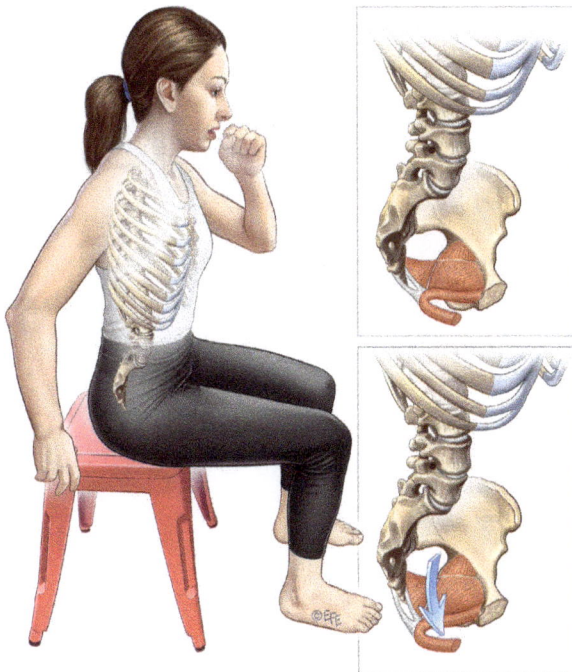

Test Two

This time sit on a chair or on the floor and cough, noticing the response in your pelvic floor muscles. Did they stay in the same position, lift or pushdown?

Your abdominal wall is the wall of your core, and your pelvic floor is the floor of your core. Both structures work together to provide continence and stability for every activity we perform, whether it is cleaning the bathroom or doing a shoulder press at the gym.

In these tests, if you feel your belly pushing out and your pelvic floor bearing down, it is a sign that your core muscles are not functioning as they should: as a *wall* and as a *floor*. They are unable to provide the support and stability demanded by the increase of IAP that in this case involves coughing.

If you have a functional core, your abdominal wall and your pelvic floor muscles prepare and engage upon an increase of IAP. So instead of pushing out they should automatically tighten without any sort of conscious activation. I'll explain more later.

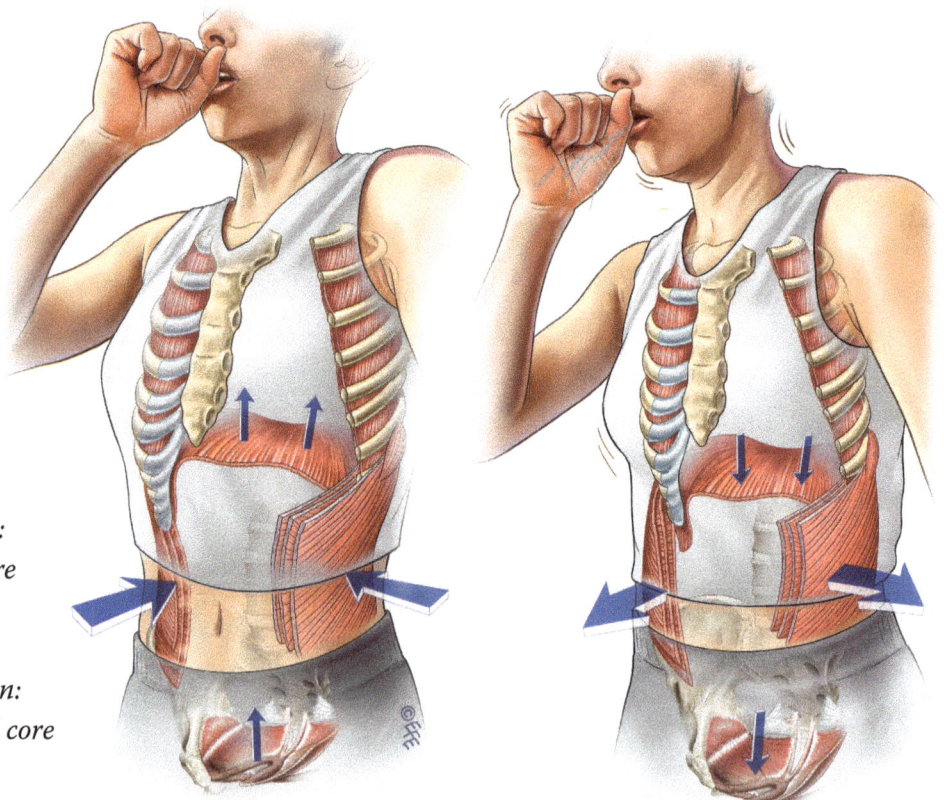

Left illustration:
A functional core
when coughing.

Right illustration:
A dysfunctional core
when coughing.

Note that, the cough test can change depending on the position. The abdominal wall can engage – for example when sitting down, but not when lying on the floor. Our goal is to make it functional in all positions and actions you perform.

THE REASON IT IS CRITICAL FOR YOUR CORE TO MANAGE IAP IS THAT IF IT DOESN'T, YOU CAN INCREASE YOUR CHANCES OF SUFFERING:

- Stress urinary incontinence

- Pelvic organ prolapse

- Disk, groin, umbilical or abdominal hernias

A normal value of IAP is 5–7 mmHg. Obesity can increase these values to 9–14 mmHg.[12]

Here are a few examples of IAP values performing different activities: [13,14]

- Scrubbing floor on hands and knees: 8.02 mmHg

- Seated shoulder press lifting 9.1 Kg: 16.04 mmHg

- Walk 4.8 Km/h 0% grade: 18.11 mmHg

- Abdominal curl ups: 16.26 mmHg

- Full sit up with feet held: 42.25 mmHg

- Jumping: 64.66 mmHg

- Coughing: 73.76 mmHg

As you can see, high-impact exercise or heavy lifting increases IAP considerably.

Overlooking the role of the core and pelvic floor in these activities could **DAMAGE** the supportive structures of your pelvis and **WEAKEN** their muscles, making them more vulnerable to **INCONTINENCE, PROLAPSE OR HERNIA.**

MUSCLE TONE: THE ANSWER TO "FLAT BELLY FRUSTRATION"

The difference between muscle strength and muscle tone can get technical, but it's essential to understand it so you can train your core correctly. We often hear and use expressions like "I need to strengthen my core", "I want to tone up my abdominals", and "I do exercises to strengthen my pelvic floor" without knowing the difference between the terms tone and strength.

We often confuse them as the same thing or sometimes refer to tone when we mean muscle definition without understanding the difference. REMEMBER THIS: your muscles can be strong but still have a low muscle tone.

Simply explained:

MUSCLE STRENGTH is the ability of a muscle to contract on command. This means that your brain voluntarily tells your muscles to contract to perform a movement. For example, lifting your baby. As your baby grows heavier, you will develop more strength to lift him or her. It's a voluntary and conscious action of the muscles regulated by the motor and sensory cortex in your brain.

MUSCLE TONE is the degree of muscle tension when it is at rest. Press your abdominals while they are relaxed; how hard do they feel? That is your abdominal tone. Muscle tone is regulated by messages from the spinal cord and the cerebellum, which means there is no conscious participation in the muscle tone. It's a combination of reflex responses and is influenced by the stiffness and flexibility of the muscular and connective tissue. Given the reflex nature of muscle tone, training to improve muscle tone it's done in a different way than to improve muscle strength.

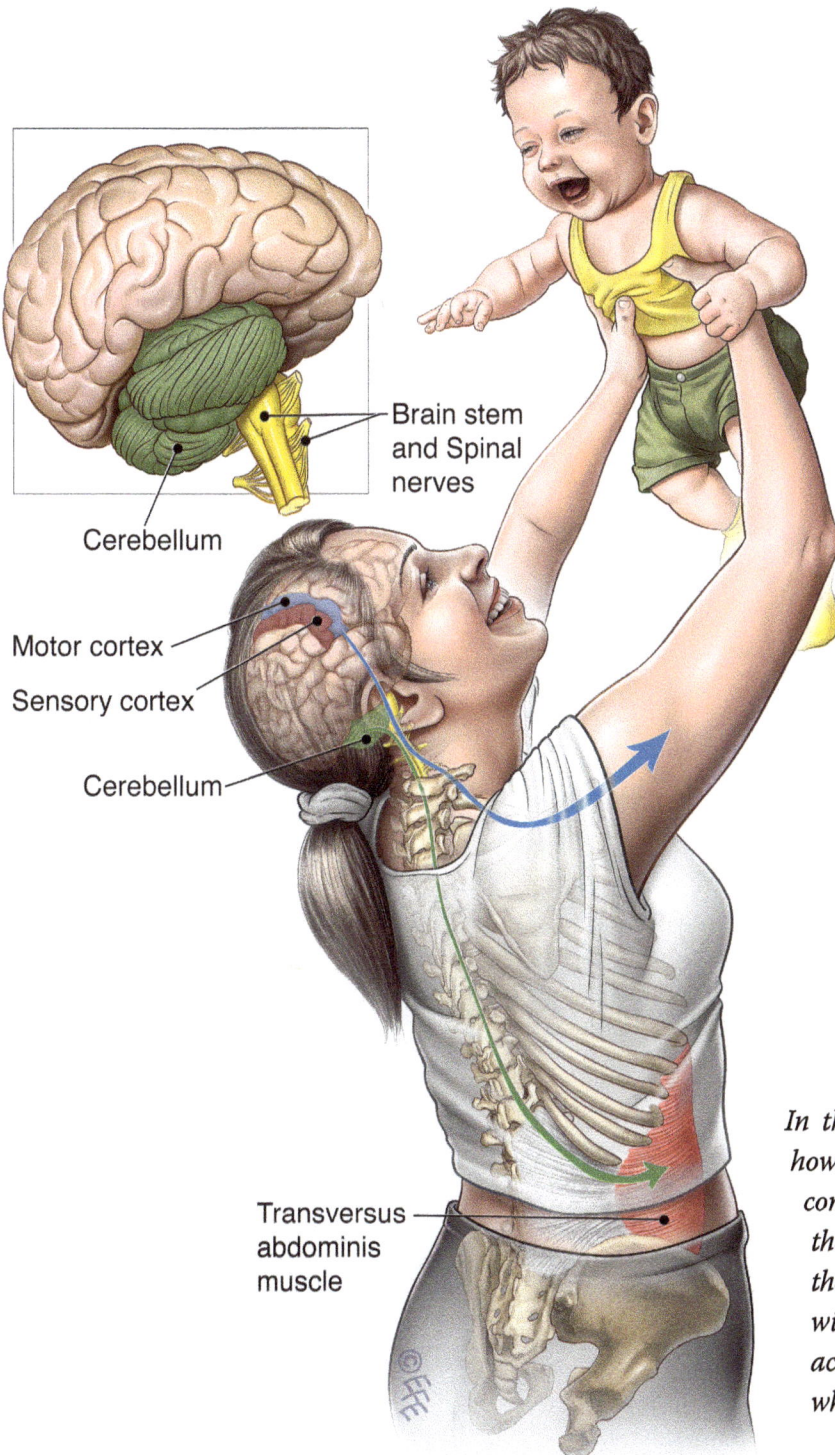

Brain stem and Spinal nerves

Cerebellum

Motor cortex

Sensory cortex

Cerebellum

Transversus abdominis muscle

In this illustration, we can see how the motor and sensory cortex control the movement of the arms to lift the baby, and the cerebellum and brain stem will regulate the core muscles activation to provide stability while performing this action.

MUSCLE TONE'S primary role is maintaining static posture, continence and stability in every movement. In contrast, MUSCLE STRENGTH is responsible for dynamic conscious movements.

FOR EXAMPLE, when you are standing, your abdominal wall is activated unconsciously to support your body and keep you upright. This is the muscle tone's role. But when you are doing crunches, you are voluntarily (consciously) contracting your core muscles and, therefore, strengthening them.

LET'S DIG A BIT DEEPER INTO THE TONE AND STRENGTH CONCEPT

Our muscles consist of fibres, of which there are two main types:

1. **TYPE I, also known as a slow twitch fibre.**
2. **TYPE II, also known as a fast twitch fibre**

All muscles have both types, but the proportion varies depending on the function the muscle develops: static/maintain posture/ stabilise or dynamic/perform movement. The main difference between the two is how they contract, and the time it takes to become fatigued.

TYPE I (slow twitch) fibres contract at a low intensity but can maintain that contraction for longer periods before becoming fatigued. That is why they exist more in muscles responsible for performing sustained or small movements and posture. Postural muscles are designed to support your body for the whole day, and even when lying down, they still show some activation.

TYPE II (fast twitch) fibres contract at a higher intensity, but fatigue more quickly. And which muscles have a higher proportion of these fibres? We use dynamic muscles to perform daily tasks and physical activity exercises.

AND WHAT IS THE RELATIONSHIP BETWEEN MUSCLE FIBRES AND MUSCLE FUNCTIONS?

- Slow twitch fibres are associated to posture and stability and they are developed through endurance training.

- Fast twitch fibres are associated to more dynamic movements and they are developed through strength training.

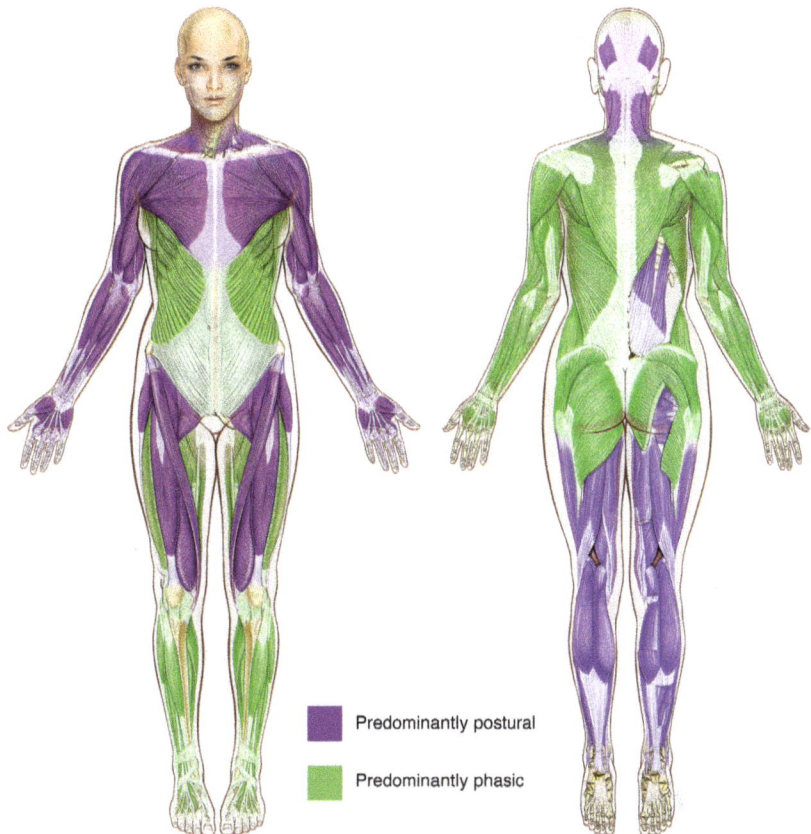

Predominantly postural

Predominantly phasic

The small and deeper muscles closer to your pelvis and spine are designed to provide support and stability and have a higher percentage of TYPE I (slow twitch) fibres. These muscles do not perform an actual movement, but they participate in stabilising the body while the movement is performed. On the other side, the large and superficial muscles that are stronger and perform voluntary movements have a higher percentage of TYPE II (fast twitch) fibres. They can also be referred to as phasic muscles.

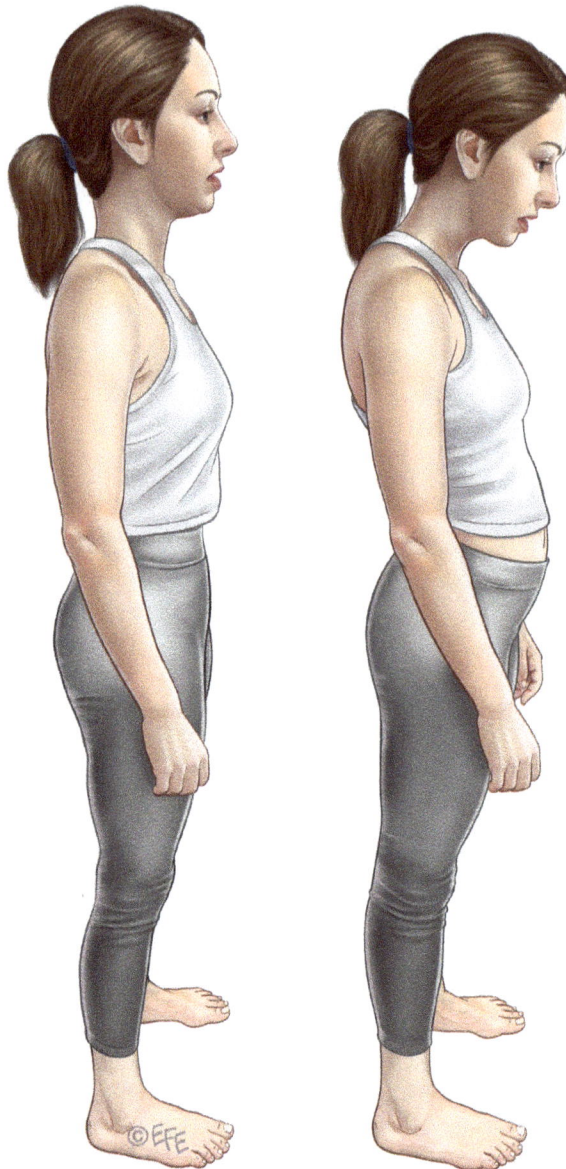

As mentioned before, your muscle tone is responsible for maintaining your posture and providing stability and continence. Low tone in the postural muscles is part of the cause of the slouch position, as you see in the image. A balanced muscle tone will keep the body in the correct alignment. You can have strong back muscles yet still have bad posture due to tone imbalances. Too high in some muscles and too low in others.

AND HOW DO TYPE I AND II FIBRES RELATE TO THE CORE AND PELVIC FLOOR TRAINING?

All core functions (stability, support, continence and breathing) must be constantly maintained throughout the day.

> For example, even when lying down, our pelvic floor muscles are still active to maintain continence. We just don't think about it because it is an unconscious reflex function of our body.

The Type I fibres (slow twitch) of your muscles are always switched on to make sure continence and support are guaranteed.

There was a study done some time ago in which they analysed the chemical composition of the muscle fibres and of some of the core muscles (internal and external obliques, transversus abdominis and rectus
abdominis) and compared them with the main pelvic floor muscle (levator ani muscle) and an arm muscle (deltoids).[15] The results showed that 2/3 of the muscle fibres of the core muscles are Type I.

This is the breakdown in percentage of Type I muscle fibres in this study:

Rectus abdominis: 69%

External obliques: 52%

Internal obliques: 69%

Levator ani muscle (pelvic floor): 55%

Deltoids (shoulder): 36%

WHAT ARE THESE RESULTS TELLING US?

That core muscles have a predominantly tonic activity. This needs to be considered when training them, as the exercises we choose will stimulate our muscle fibres differently.

Will performing crunches, planks and all those exercises at the gym strengthen your core muscles?

Yes, but they will not necessarily make your belly flat.

Will performing pelvic floor clenching exercises improve your pelvic floor muscle strength?

Yes, but they will not necessarily permanently fix your incontinence and prolapse symptoms.

The reflect activation of the core muscles can "go a bit silent" after pregnancy, birth, continuous heavy weight lifting, high impact exercises or just simply the ageing process. Although initially we can help restore it by consciously activating the muscles, the goal is to establish the reflex activation. This can be achieved with a more complete and holistic training approach that also involves breathing and the postural aspects that help create a synergistic activation of your core muscles involuntarily. We will discuss this later in the book.

WHAT HAPPENS WHEN WE HAVE TOO MUCH MUSCLE TONE (HYPERTONIA)?

Too much tone isn't good for your core, either. Constant activation of the pelvic floor and abdominal muscles can lead to HYPERTONIA, when these muscles cannot relax and therefore restrict blood flow and neural function.

Hypertonia is often related to pelvic or back pain, inability to void (urinary retention), painful sex and difficulties during labour.

Unsupervised pelvic floor strength training can have terrible consequences for someone with an overactive pelvic floor, as it can worsen the problem and become painful. Imagine severe neck pain in your pelvis!

Constant abdominal bracing can also lead to hypertonia. In fact, abdominal bracing increases intra-abdominal pressure, which can interfere with bowel movements and aggravate symptoms of prolapse or incontinence.

If you think you have symptoms of hypertonicity of your pelvic floor or abdominal muscles, it is important to visit a physiotherapist specialising in pelvic floor disorders to get an accurate diagnosis and appropriate treatment.

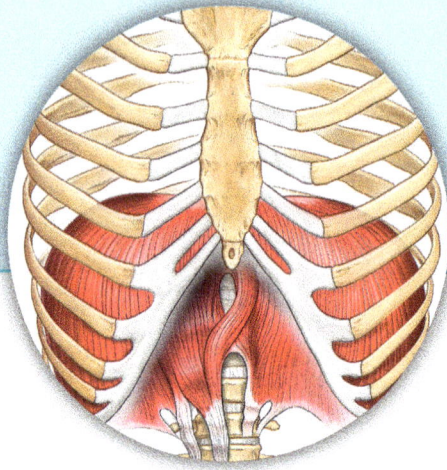

HOW YOU STAND AND BREATH
MATTERS

03

HOW YOU STAND AND BREATHE MATTERS

POSTURE AND BREATHING PATTERNS
HAVE AN **IMPACT** ON YOUR CORE AND PELVIC FLOOR FUNCTION

Critical aspects of our core and pelvic floor health that are usually not considered is our posture and breathing patterns.

> GOOD POSTURAL ALIGNMENT CONTRIBUTES NOT ONLY TO OPTIMAL BIOMECHANICAL FUNCTION BUT TO THE HEALTHY FUNCTIONING OF ORGANS.

As I mentioned earlier, muscles do not work independently. For example, when you do an abdominal crunch, muscles other than the rectus abdominis (six-pack) participate in the action. Muscles are also connected by fascia, a web of connective tissue that wraps muscles together. This plays an important role in supporting the body and assisting with movements.

For example, when you roll your spine down to reach your toes, you probably feel tightness throughout different parts of the back section of your body. You can feel it in the back of your legs, around the spine or even in the neck. This action stretches all the muscles located at the back of your body and the fascia holding them together.

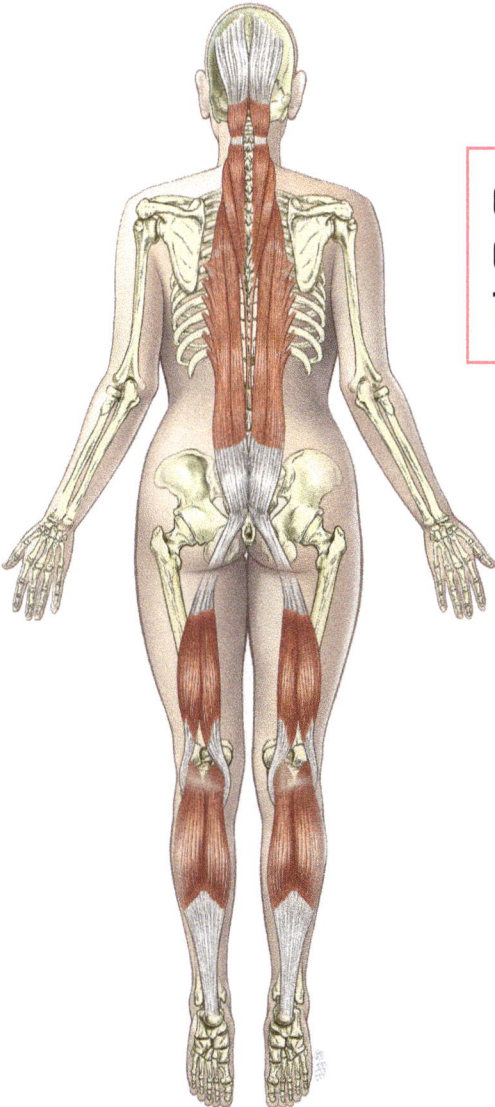

The muscular and fascial chain at the back of the body plays an essential role in keeping us standing upright.

The fascia relies on the concept of tensegrity (tension + integrity), which is how the different tensile forces of the body maintain the body's structural shape. Figuratively speaking, your body behaves like a camping tent. The different poles and ropes keep it up, and if you tense one of the ropes too much, it will tilt to one side. Our muscles, bones, ligaments and fascia respond similarly: when continuous tension is applied to one part of the body, different structures adapt to that stimulus. This is why an old ankle sprain can cause unexplained neck pain months, or even years, later.

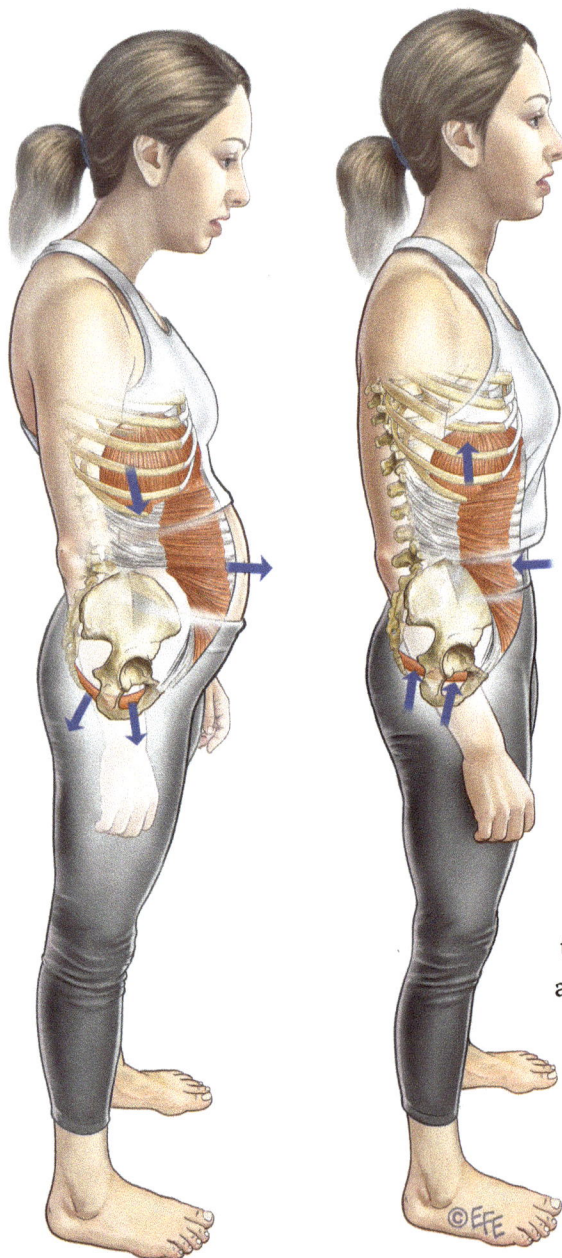

> Maintaining a balance in the tensions of the body keeps it in good ALIGNMENT and has a significant and positive effect on your core and pelvic function.

Posture affects intra-abdominal pressure, as shown in the image, and is linked to pelvic floor function. Just by improving static posture, you will reduce the pressure on your core and pelvic floor. Additionally, your stomach should flatten thanks to the tension in your muscles and fascia of your abdominal wall.

GOOD CORE FUNCTION STARTS WITH GOOD POSTURE!

HOW POSTURE AND BREATHING CONNECT

Your physical posture also affects your breathing. The way you sit, stand and hold yourself can restrict your breathing. Abdominal bracing, a common practice in core training, limits free-flowing breathing by tightening abdominal muscles. You can experience it yourself by bracing your stomach muscles and trying to inhale deeply. You probably had to lift your shoulders to get adequate air into your lungs. When the chest muscles are used, it is known as shallow breathing, and predominantly chest breathing is a common cause of neck pain and headaches. This is another reason excessive tone in the abdominal wall can be counterproductive.

Our daily habits also impact our posture. Computers, mobile phones and jobs that involve sitting for long periods cause us to slouch; our shoulders roll forward and our head tilts down. This also restricts our breathing.

Try this simple exercise to realise how much the alignment of the head can affect breathing:

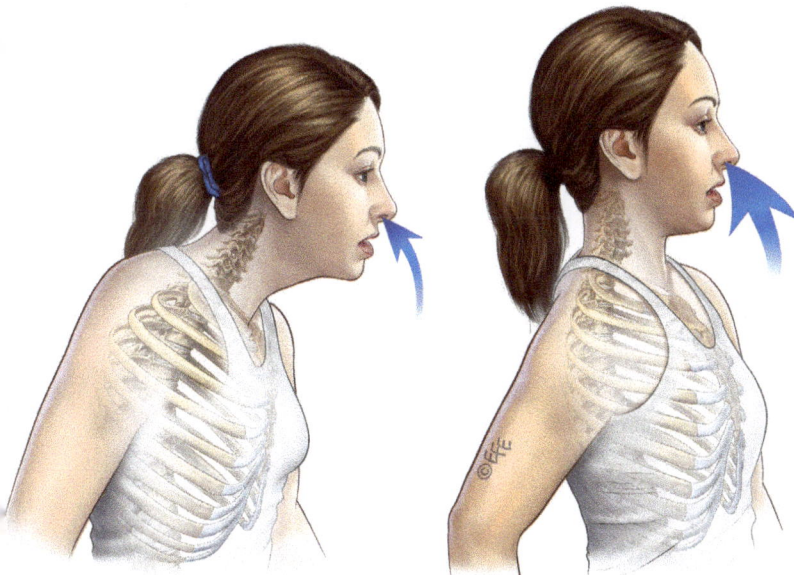

1. Stand with your head tilted forward and try to breathe deeply. Notice how it feels. *(left image)*

2. Now, tuck your chin in, bringing your head in alignment to a neutral position. Elongate your neck and breathe in deeply. Now notice how it feels. *(right image)*

You probably found it much harder to breathe with your head forward than in correct alignment.

The alignment of our pelvis and ribcage also impacts our breathing parameters. A study has found that when the pelvis and the ribcage are aligned correctly in a neutral position, certain breathing parameters are much better.[16] Along with other muscles in the body, core muscles keep the neutral position of the pelvis and the ribcage.

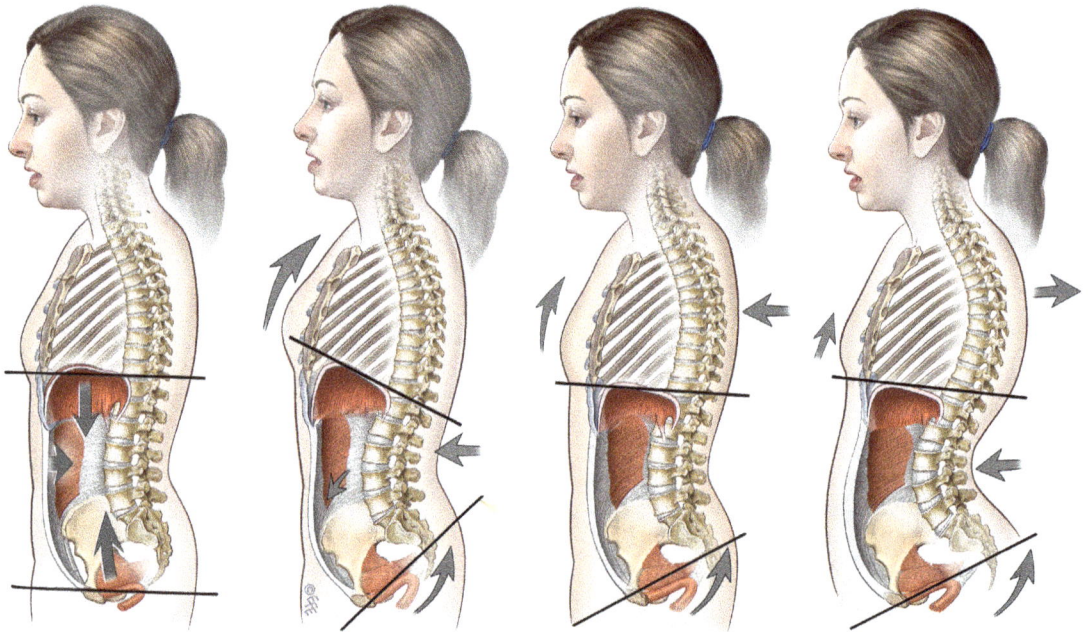

Another interesting study shows the effect that the positioning of the foot and ankle have on pelvic floor activation: Dorsiflexion of the ankle induces changes to the pelvic floor muscles attachments and the positioning of the sacrum and coccyx allows these muscles to activate better than when the ankle is in plantar flexion.

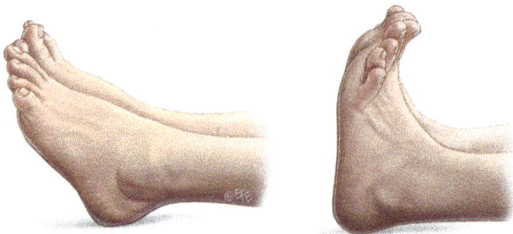

The study suggests that women with stress urinary incontinence should be discouraged from wearing high heel shoes as it can damage the pelvic floor.[17]

Plantar flexion left illustration, Dorsiflexion right)

HOW THE PELVIC FLOOR AND BREATHING CONNECT

Most people are unaware of how poor breathing can negatively affect their pelvic floor. To understand how we breathe, we need to know how the diaphragm works.

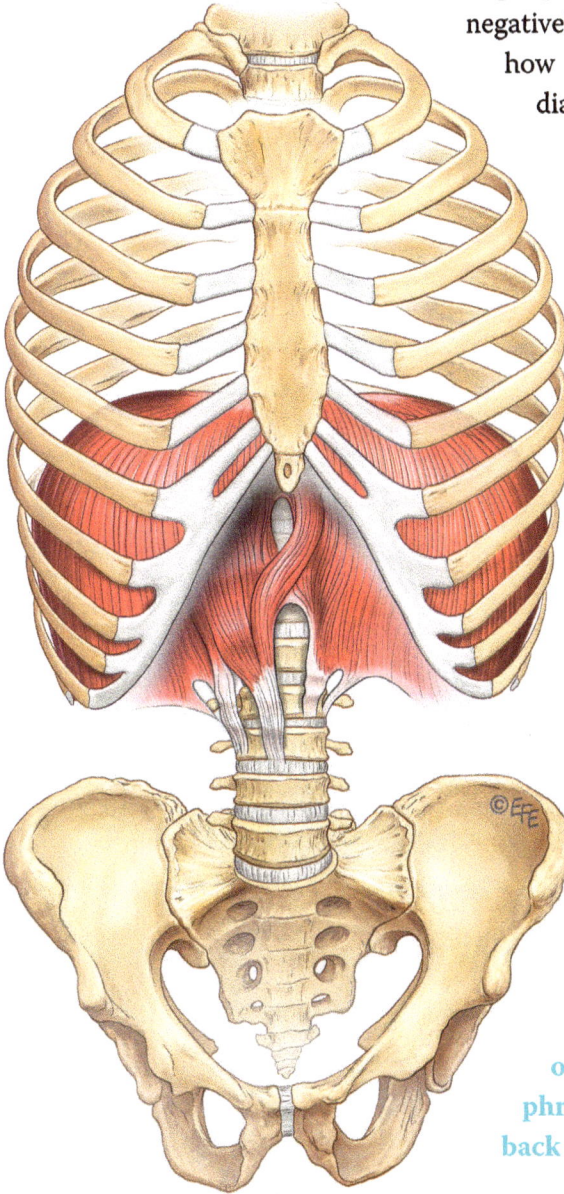

The diaphragm *(in the image)* is the dome-shaped muscle located in the midsection of the body. It separates the lungs and heart from the abdominal cavity and is anchored across the ribs and the lumbar vertebrae. It has three orifices to allow the vena cava, the aorta artery (the blood vessels that come into and out of the heart) and the oesophagus to pass through it. As well as the vagus nerve that regulates the function of many organs located in your abdominal cavity.

The diaphragm is constantly working, contracting and relaxing with our breathing, and just like calf muscles can get tight after a long run, your diaphragm does too.

A tight diaphragm will restrict breathing capacity and, therefore, the supply of oxygen to our bodies. An overly tight diaphragm can negatively impact posture, cause back pain and affect your pelvic floor.

DIAPHRAGMATIC BREATHING

Is when you mainly use your diaphragm, letting the air fill the bottom of your lungs and expand your ribs and belly rather than using the accessory muscles around your neck and upper chest. We are born breathing like this but tend to lose this pattern as we age due to stress, pregnancy, poor ergonomics and repetitive movements.

SHALLOW BREATHING

Is when you draw the air into the chest area instead of the bottom of the lungs. This means minimal air is taken into the lungs, and intercostal and neck muscles are mainly used to expand the chest area. Shallow breathing can impact pelvic floor dysfunction. If the ribs lift during inhalation and then drop during exhalation, they force the abdominal wall outwards and the pelvic floor downwards.

The pelvic floor is sometimes referred to as the pelvic diaphragm. The muscles and tissues in your pelvic region form a hammock that provides trunk stabilisation and keeps your internal organs in place. Your pelvic diaphragm, part of your core, also has fascial connections to your abdominal muscles and breathing diaphragm. These all move in sync when we breathe and move.

The synergistic activation of the pelvic floor muscles and transversus has been demonstrated in electromyography studies[18] ELECTROMYOGRAPHY is a technnique used to identify and assess the electrical activity in the muscles. This same procedure has been used to find out that the surrounding abdominal muscles optimise pelvic floor contraction.[19]

THIS IS THE WAY YOUR CORE STRUCTURES MOVE DURING NORMAL BREATHING:[20]

ON THE INHALATION

(Left image), your diaphragm contracts, making it descend (allowing space for your lungs to expand) and the abdominal wall moves out, as a result of the internal organs being pushed by the diaphragm. And your pelvic floor descends slightly.

ON THE EXHALATION

(Right image), your diaphragm rises pushing the air out of the lungs. Your abdominal wall moves in towards your spine, and your pelvic floor rises slightly.

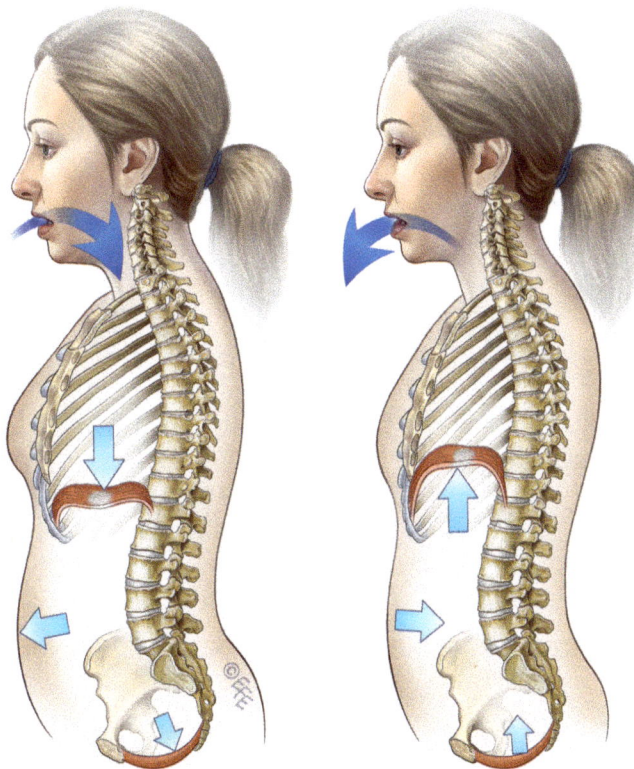

When you breathe more intensely, for example, when you cough, laugh or during exercise, these structures move in and out further. During a forced exhalation, you can feel your abdominal muscles tighten. They are called "expiratory muscles" because they actively participate in the exhalation phase of the breathing cycle.

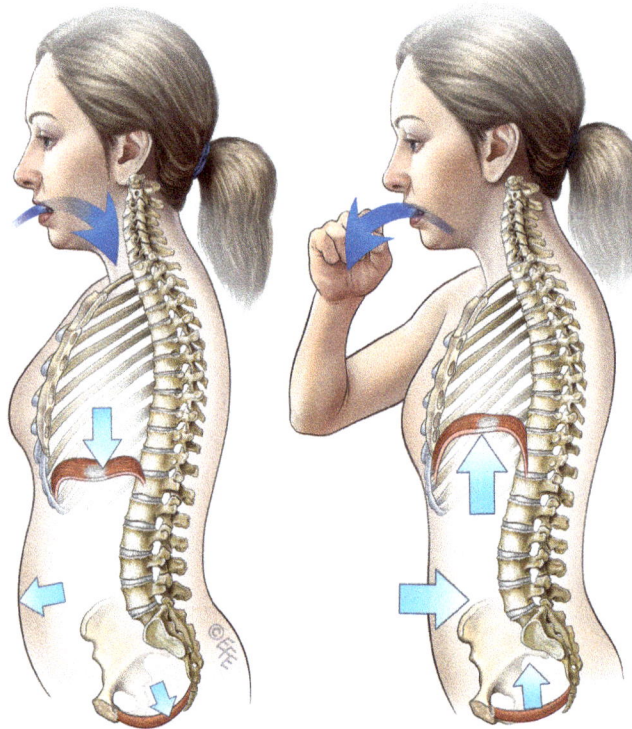

Coughing and sneezing are just strong exhalations, meaning the core structures should respond the same way as the images above. But when the core is dysfunctional, the abdominal wall and pelvic floor move in the opposite direction that they should in the exhalation phase, pushing out instead of engaging and drawing in.

There are so many BENEFITS to be had by learning to breathe correctly.

See below the image to the left during the inhalation phase, and to the right the incorrect exhalation pattern where the abdominal wall and pelvic floor move outwards.

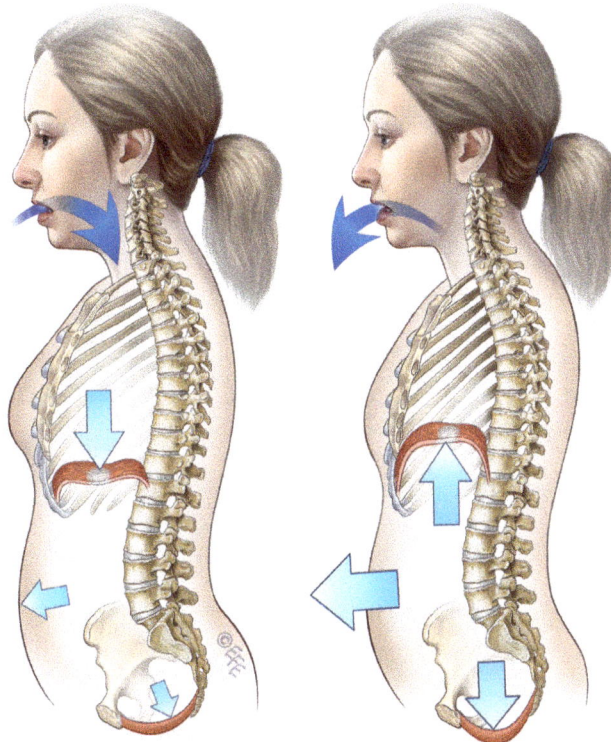

Correct breathing will not only improve your core and pelvic floor, but it will also improve your overall health:

- As your chest becomes more relaxed, so do your neck and shoulders, reducing pain.

- The correct movement of your diaphragm massages your internal organs (liver, stomach and intestines), facilitating their function.

- Better diaphragmatic mobility improves blood and lymphatic circulation.

- Breathing with the diaphragm induces relaxation and reduces anxiety by modulating your sympathetic and parasympathetic systems.

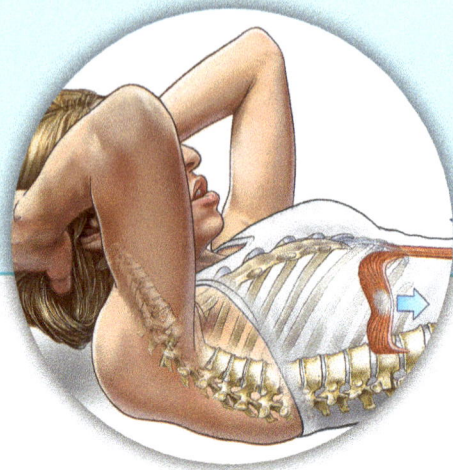

CHAPTER 04

STRESS URINARY INCONTINENCE (SUI), THE SILENT EPIDEMIC

NOTE

This chapter refers exclusively to STRESS URINARY INCONTINENCE and its relationship to core training and physical activity. Different types of urinary incontinence can be related to other health problems, so please refer to your doctor if you have any concerns about your bladder or bowel control.

04 STRESS URINARY INCONTINENCE (SUI), THE SILENT EPIDEMIC

EXERCISING WITH AN **INCONTINENCE** PAD DOES NOT FIX THE PROBLEM

STRESS URINARY INCONTINENCE

Although rarely spoken about, stress urinary incontinence is a world-wide health issue that mostly affects women, although some men experience it too.

Incontinence is not a life-threatening condition, but you shouldn't have to live with it.

It causes embarrassment and, in some cases, can impact someone's lifestyle so much that they suffer from depression.

Unfortunately, there is a lack of information about it, with many sufferers having no idea what to do to fix it.

WHAT IS IT?

Stress urinary incontinence is the involuntary leakage of urine when performing a physical movement or actions like laughing, coughing or blowing your nose.

To maintain continence, we need our pelvic floor and core muscles to work against the increased intra-abdominal pressure. When they are weak and/or not working in sync, the pressure on the bladder produced by a specific activity is higher than the pressure on the sphincter and cannot maintain continence.

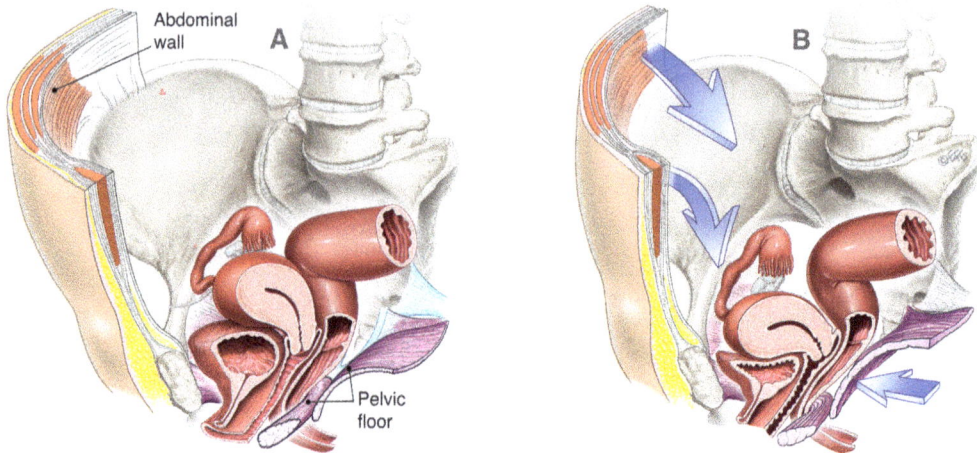

Abdominal wall

A

B

Pelvic floor

Left illustration shows the normal positioning of the bladder, uterus and rectum. Right illustration shows how an increase in intra-abdominal pressure can provoke a descent of the organs in the pelvic cavity into the bladder.

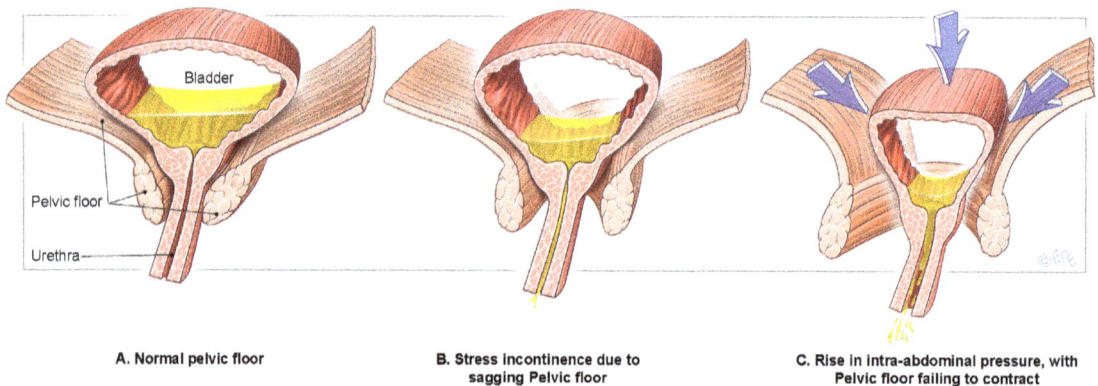

Bladder

Pelvic floor

Urethra

A. Normal pelvic floor

B. Stress incontinence due to sagging Pelvic floor

C. Rise in intra-abdominal pressure, with Pelvic floor failing to contract

Many people with SIU regard it as normal when it is simply common. Experiencing urinary leakage when you cough or sneeze is NOT normal. Wearing a pad when exercising or avoiding exercise because of leakage is NOT normal. And crossing your legs to prevent leakage before sneezing is NOT normal.

This condition can be treated; you can save a lot of money on incontinence pads and invest it in a good therapist that can prescribe you the right exercises for a long-term solution.

TWO ASPECTS ARE CONSIDERED RELEVANT IN SUI AND CORE:

1. Lack of muscle tone means the at-rest tension in your pelvic floor muscles is low, and you are unable to manage increased pressure while performing an activity.

2. Lack of synergy in your core muscles means your pelvic floor muscles don't move in sync with your abdominal wall and diaphragm to modulate the pressure produced by the action performed.

There are many factors involved in the possible causes of SUI. The most common is the effects of pregnancy and delivery that can cause damage to the muscular, connective or neural tissues or even the actual urinary tract. But the effects of ageing can also impact incontinence as well as obesity and high-impact and strenuous physical activity.

STRESS URINARY INCONTINENCE AND PHYSICAL ACTIVITY: THE WORKOUT PEE

Urinary incontinence is more common in older women, but young women can have it too. In the past fifty years, the number of women engaged in regular physical activity and competitive sports has increased dramatically. You probably never saw your grandmother going to the gym every week to do a weightlifting session, but now it's common to see women practising CrossFit, running marathons or competing in boxing, for example. Our lifestyle has changed, and women have become more present in sports and fitness.

This is great, but unfortunately, this trend coincides with a disturbingly high occurrence of SUI in women, even amongst young women who have not experienced childbirth yet.[21] I love that women are exercising and competing, but given the high prevalence of SUI, shouldn't we consider if we are doing something wrong? A possible explanation is that the repetitive increase in intra-abdominal pressure can lead to weakness and stretching of the pelvic floor muscles and, consequently, to urinary incontinence and damage the pelvic area's connective tissues and ligaments.[22] So, sports involving more jumping can put you at a higher risk of incontinence. However, low-impact sports such as swimming still have a 15% prevalence of incontinence and Yoga and Pilates instructors also report a prevalence of 25.9%. This could be explained by the constant demand for spinal stability that can provoke urinary alterations.[23] Below is a table showing the prevalence of urinary incontinence amongst female athletes in different sports.[22]

Sport	Total of athletes assessed	Number of athletes reporting urinary incontinence	Prevalence %
Basketball	45	19	42.22%
Football	38	19	50.00%
Gymnastics	371	227	61.19%
Tennis	6	3	50.00%
Volleyball	139	80	57.55%
Hockey	19	6	31.58%
Judo	9	4	44.44%
Running	635	197	31.02%
Softball	16	1	6.25%
Track and field	63	1	6.25%
Bodybuilding	164	23	14.02%
Cycling	89	8	10.11%
Hiking	99	12	12.12%
Pilates	36	2	5.56%
Swimming	118	18	12.64%

Peeing during a workout is not a badge of honour but a sign of weakness and core dysfunction. Wearing pads or special underwear or emptying your bladder before exercising does not fix the problem; many people stop exercising because of urine loss, or change the type of physical activity or just walk to reduce urinary symptoms.[24] This doesn't fix the problem either, as regular exercise is vital to maintain general health and stopping would only bring more issues.

There is no such thing as bad exercise; we just need to be aware of the effects of some forms of physical activity on our core's integrity and take action to correctly exercise our core so we can continue doing the activities we love. Correct core and pelvic floor training will allow you to keep active for life without embarrassment.

A MESSAGE FOR PARENTS OF YOUNG ATHLETES

I came across clients whose daughters were participating in competitive sports at a high level during my career. After learning about pelvic and core health, they became aware that their young daughters could potentially suffer SUI from the high-impact actions involved in their sports.

SUI at a young age can occur in sports like gymnastics, for example, as we have already seen. There are studies where young athletes complained about the sporadic loss of small quantities of urine; however, they showed no symptoms during their training routine.[25]

There is not enough information about long-term urinary symptoms in athletes and what happens after they stop competitive training compared to those who haven't practised high-impact sports at a competitive level. The existing studies show different results; the most reliable theory is that strenuous exercises may prompt the early onset of incontinence symptoms that would appear later in life in predisposed women.

Therefore, women should start prevention as soon as they start exercising.[25–27]

And this can be done by including exercises targeted to maintain a healthy core function and breathing patterns and specific pelvic floor muscle training in the training programs. The exercises explained at the end of this book will help prevent the injuries and dysfunctions high-impact physical activities can cause.

WHY CONVENTIONAL SIT-UPS AND CRUNCHES COULD BE MAKING YOU MORE INCONTINENT

Whenever you perform an action that curls your spine, you compress the organs in your abdominal and pelvic cavity. The upper body pushes your internal organs towards your abdomen and pelvic floor, overwhelming these muscles. Constant repetition of this action will result in a loss of tone and, consequently, an incapacity to control (close) your sphincter muscles unless you consciously clench them.

This illustration shows it well:

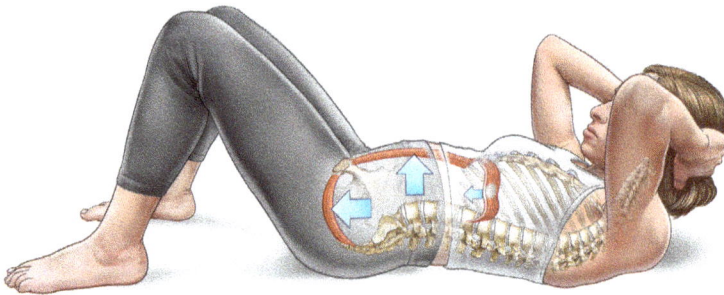

In the FIRST IMAGE, you can see the intra-abdominal pressure push against the weakest parts of your core, those not protected by bone; your abdominal wall and pelvic floor.

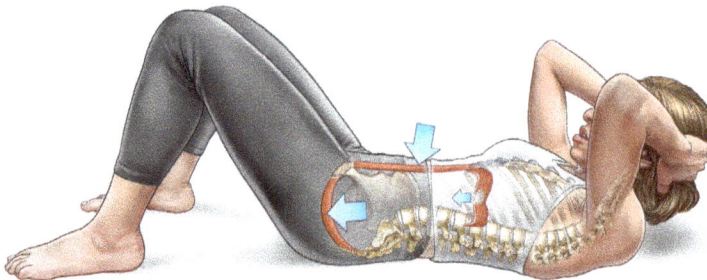

In the SECOND IMAGE, a crunch is performed while bracing the abdominal wall, preventing it from bulging out during the action. In this case, all the pressure moves in one direction, towards the pelvic floor.

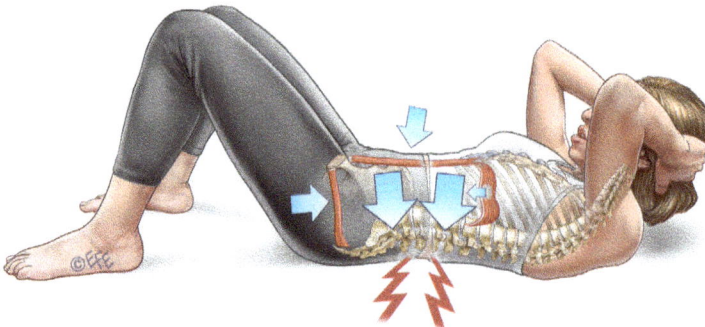

In the THIRD IMAGE, the same action is performed while activating the abdominal wall and pelvic floor. This moves the pressure to the spine and can cause back pain and even disc injuries.

Some studies show that this

type of exercise can increase intra-abdominal pressure and bladder depression in both continent and incontinent women.[28,29]

This must be considered, when designing a core training program for women.

WHAT ABOUT PLANKS?

Planks are often prescribed by professionals as a safer alternative to crunches. Although there is no curling when you plank, it still increases your intra-abdominal pressure, which can still impact any weak area of your core. (People often complain of back pain while doing planks). Planks can be adapted in many ways to the person's fitness level and conditions. Still, gentle postural exercises and breathing techniques that activate your deep core muscles should be practised before starting plank exercises to build a functional core foundation.

TREATING STRESS URINARY INCONTINENCE

Kegel exercises are normally the first treatment line for SUI, a series of pelvic floor muscle contractions performed at different intensities and durations designed to improve their strength. The problem is that these voluntary contractions of the pelvic floor can be hard to perform because the muscles are inside the pelvis where we cannot see them, making it difficult to identify them. Additionally, they are very small.

> To perform Kegels correctly, it is important to make sure you lift your pelvic floor muscles rather than contracting others, such as your adductors or gluteus.

If you want to learn to "Kegel" correctly, I highly recommend you visit a pelvic floor physiotherapist who can teach you how to identify and engage these muscles. Also, when the pelvic floor is hypertonic, Kegel exercises are contraindicated, so it's important to get properly assessed by a pelvic therapist to determine whether these exercises are suitable or not.

Kegel exercises are part of the foundation for a healthy pelvic floor;

however you will also need to improve your posture and breathing patterns to have a fully functional core and overcome SUI. This is what research says about it:

- When the ability of the transverse abdominis muscle to contract is impaired, it negatively affects pelvic floor muscles and consequently increases the risk of urinary incontinence.[18,30]

- If we relax the abdominal wall during pelvic floor muscle contraction, we will be reaching only 25% of the maximal capacity of contraction of the pelvic floor.[31]

- By improving the coordination of the diaphragm with the abdominal wall and pelvic floor muscles, we will likely reduce stress urinary incontinence by optimising the expiratory patterns[20,31].

When you have ongoing back pain that restricts your daily activities and reduces your quality of life, the norm is to get a diagnosis and an appropriate treatment so you can get back to your normal

> **STRESS URINARY INCONTINENCE NEEDS TO BE CONSIDERED AS A MUSCULO-SKELETAL INJURY OR WEAKNESS**

life as soon as possible. Likewise, urinary incontinence is your pelvic floor screaming for help – you need to do something about it!

Talk to your doctor and visit a therapist specialising in pelvic floor disorders. There is nothing embarrassing about it; pelvic floor muscles are just the floor of your core, a collection of muscles you want to look after.

Your therapist will be able to give you a proper diagnosis and the most appropriate treatment for you. And do not wait until the problem escalates; even a minimal leak is a sign of weakness! The sooner you take action, the quicker and easier treating it will be.

SOME HELPFUL NOTES REGARDING STRESS URINARY INCONTINENCE

- Be aware that impact activities and heavy lifting can weaken the pelvic floor, so make sure you include pelvic floor training in your regular exercise routine to keep the muscles functioning correctly and maintain continence.

- Whenever you perform an exercise that increases considerably IAP, such as lifting a weight (including lifting your children). **EXHALE during exertion! Try not to hold your breath.**

- Chronic coughing or sneezing can weaken your pelvic floor and cause incontinence, so ask your doctor for the best treatment for your condition.

- Healthy toilet habits: Bearing down while urinating and defecating adds pressure to your pelvic floor and organs, so take your time in the toilet and let gravity do its job. Avoid constipation by drinking plenty of fluids and eating fruits and vegetables rich in fibre and consider using a toilet stool (squat potty) to aid complete defecation.

- Do not hold on to urine. Make sure you go to the toilet when you feel the urge to urinate.

- Diabetes can increase the urge to urinate. If you have diabetes, keep your sugar levels under control and avoid processed foods and sugar.

- Keep in mind that alcohol and caffeinated drinks increase the urge to urinate, and spicy foods, carbonated drinks and citrus can also irritate the bladder. If you are experiencing urinary leakage, try to reduce your consumption of these.

- Smoking increases bladder irritation and the risk of bladder cancer. Consider quitting.

- An excess of fat in the abdominal area can increase the pressure on your bladder, so losing weight can reduce your chances of incontinence.

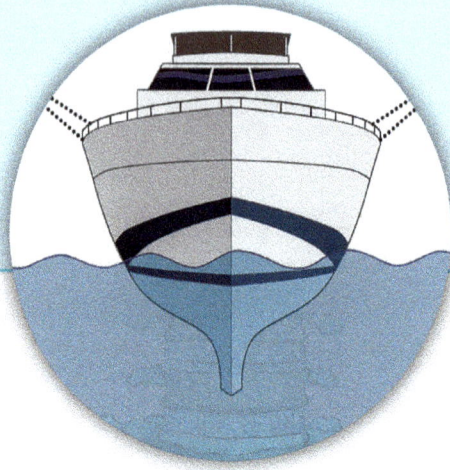

CHAPTER 05

PELVIC ORGAN PROLAPSE, YOU'RE NOT ALONE

05

PELVIC ORGAN PROLAPSE, YOU'RE NOT ALONE

BY THE TIME WOMEN REACH THEIR 80'S, HALF OF THEM WILL SUFFER FROM PROLAPSE

I first heard about prolapse when I was a personal trainer. Prolapse is when the bladder, uterus or bowel drops down into the vagina ('pro-lapse' literally means to 'fall out of place'). I researched it extensively and realised that my training programs could aggravate it. I was horri-fied that my clients might silently suffer while I made them jump with a skipping rope, sprint, or do V crunches.

By the time most women learn about pelvic organ prolapse they already suffer symptoms. Many women, desperate to get their pre-baby body back, rush into old exercise habits as soon as they get the green light. Thinking they can just do the same as they used to and then one day, suddenly, something feels unpleasantly different.

It may start by feeling like a tampon is falling out, as if you were sitting on a golf ball or even just a sense of heaviness in your pelvic area. You may have been told that is a normal change after pregnancy until you reach for a mirror to see what is happening 'below the belt' and are shocked and you wonder why no one told you this could happen. Prolapse quickly dictates every aspect of your life; it causes you pain, affects your relationships, enormously restricts your exercise options and reduces your quality of life in general.

Pelvic organ prolapse is often known as 'POP', which is the exact feeling many women experience — as if something has POPPED OUT OF THE VAGINA. Even though roughly 50% of women experience it after childbirth, it is hardly ever discussed and only addressed with a doctor when the problem notably affects the quality of life.

A good way to understand the role of the muscles and connective tissue in a pelvic organ prolapse is by looking at "the boat in dry dock" analogy explained by Professor Peggy Norton.[32] Looking at the image below, the ship represents the pelvic organs (uterus, bladder, rectum), the moorings are the ligaments and connective tissue that maintain these organs in place, and the water is the pelvic floor muscles.

When there is plenty of water in the dock (a strong pelvic floor), the boat is floating perfectly, and the moorings just hold it in place. But if we reduce the amount of water in the dock (a weak pelvic floor), it will put the moorings under a lot of strain, and if this strain is maintained for an extended period, the moorings will eventually become damaged.

When weak pelvic floor muscles fail to provide enough support, your pelvic organs respond in the same way. The connective tissue and ligaments that were supposed to *assist* become the *main support* for the pelvic organs and eventually overstrain and fail to hold the pelvic organs up. This is why it's so essential to maintain your pelvic floor tone; it provides constant support and continence to the pelvic organs.

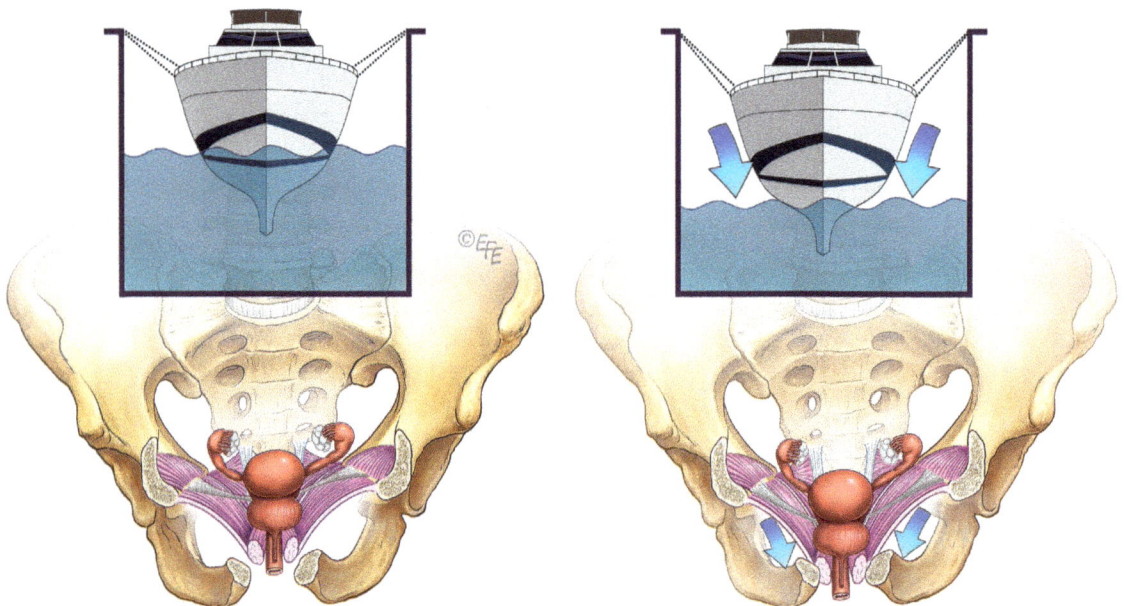

The initial symptoms usually go unnoticed; a feeling of heaviness in the pelvic area or as if something is stuck in the vaginal entrance. Other common symptoms are:

- Stress urinary incontinence

- Difficulty in emptying your bladder

- Ongoing urinary tract infections

- Tampons fall out (you are unable to keep a tampon in the vagina)

- Pain or discomfort during intercourse

> **Every woman should be educated about POP and the factors that INCREASE THE RISK of occurring before, during and after childbirth.**

The more knowledge we have, the better we can decrease (and hopefully prevent) the risk of having it. Prolapse is not something women 'just have to live with'. If you suspect you may have a prolapse, or have any of the above symptoms, visit your gynaecologist or a therapist specialising in women's health.

The most common risk factors of prolapse are:

- Changes associated with pregnancy and birth, due to the increase in progesterone production, the tissues become lax in allowing uterus expansion and increased mobility in the different structures of the pelvic area.

- Childbirth complications such as large babies, use of forceps or suction, prolonged second-stage labour, episiotomies or multiple births.

- Hormonal changes during menopause that affect the strength and elasticity of the supportive structures of the pelvic organs (muscles, ligaments and connective tissue).

- Heavy lifting and heavy weights training.

- High-impact exercise like running, jumping, skipping etc.

- Chronic coughing.

- Chronic constipation.

- Genetics: a history of POP in the family increases the likelihood of having it.[33]

- Connective tissue disorders such as Ehlers-Danos syndrome or Marfan's syndrome.

HOW TO PREVENT A PROLAPSE OR STOP IT FROM BECOMING WORSE?

Often women with prolapse develop a fear of movement because they get told to stop any form of strenuous activity, including not lifting their babies, something I consider unrealistic. They also struggle to perform daily tasks when standing up for long hours due to the effect of gravity on their pelvic organs and the lack of support.

For some women with prolapse, standing up at the end of the day to cook dinner for the family can be exhausting and very frustrating. The impact that prolapses can have on the quality of life is so high that it often leads to depression.

There is a genetic predisposition to suffer from prolapse, however; there are things that you can do to help prevent it or manage the symptoms. The first thing you need to do is get properly diagnosed by a specialist to determine the type of prolapse you have and the grade of severity, as well as monitor your symptoms.

It's important to stay active and choose the right exercises that won't aggravate your symptoms

> I HIGHLY RECOMMEND EXERCISING UNDER THE SUPERVISION OF A PROFESSIONAL WITH KNOWLEDGE OF THIS CONDITION.

by adapting the level of impact and load. Intra-abdominal pressure and gravity both increase and aggravate POP, so the exercises you do must help with both.

FOCUS ON:

- Reducing excess abdominal and visceral fat (it places pressure on your pelvic structures). A healthy diet and regular exercise are essential.

- Managing conditions related to chronic coughing or sneezing, such as smoking and allergies.

- Learning with your therapist how to engage your pelvic floor and core muscles along with breathing and be able to recreate this pattern during physical activity and daily tasks.

- Swapping activities like running or jumping for others with less impact, such as swimming, cross-trainer or bicycle.

- Reducing the load of your weights. You can still work pretty hard with low weights and elastic bands.

- Choosing positions where your body is more supported or under less gravitational strain (seated/lying instead of standing up).

- Reducing the depths of exercises like squats/lunges keeping your hips always above knee level and keep your feet hip width apart.

- Always exhale during the effort instead of holding your breath, and engage your core muscles simultaneously without bracing.

- Including in your regular training exercises that improve your posture and breathing patterns, restore the core and pelvic floor function and help manage intra-abdominal pressure the increases. The exercises included in the last chapters of this book are designed to improve these aspects.

TREATMENT OPTIONS FOR PELVIC ORGAN PROLAPSE

Make sure you have a good diet and a healthy lifestyle and follow the above recommendations. On top of that, INTRA-VAGINAL PESSARIES are a non-surgical treatment for prolapse. Pessaries are removable devices that are designed to support the herniated pelvic structures. See your pelvic floor specialist for advice about whether a pessary suits you and, if so, which size and shape will be best.

SURGERY may be an option to consider when the prolapse is severe, and all the other treatments are not enough. A doctor specialising in gynaecological surgery will explain the different procedures available and which are the most suitable ones. Be aware that current surgical techniques do not guarantee complete recovery, and you will likely need additional procedures in the future.[34]

ESTROGEN HORMONES are believed to reduce the thinning of the pelvic and vaginal tissues as it affects collagen content. Although there is no clear evidence that estrogens work, they are often used in conjunction with pessaries, pelvic floor muscle training and before or after prolapse surgery.[35]

The use of COLLAGEN in the treatment of pelvic organ prolapse has been increasing in recent years. Given the structure of the collagen surrounding the pelvic organs is loose in women suffering from prolapse,[36] there is a belief that the intake of collagen supplements can help recover the supportive capacity of the collagen in the area. However, this is based on studies made mostly in the treatment of joint health, which suggests that the ingestion of collagen peptides along with exercise could be beneficial for managing degenerative bone and joint disorders.[37]

Collagen is a protein produced in the body; inside the body cells, the DNA sequence creates the different amino acids that form the collagen protein. The synthesis of collagen is a complex process that also requires the presence of vitamin C. The production of collagen in the body starts to decrease around 25 years old. There are external factors such as smoking or sun exposure that can affect your collagen synthesis, as well as genetic factors. We also know that there is a higher prevalence of musculoskeletal injuries in women compared to males, and there is a reason to believe that female sex hormones may alter collagen protein synthesis.[38]

There are different types of collagens, and their composition is different in the skin, cartilage, tendons, ligaments, fascia, etc. The collagen present in the connective tissue inside the pelvic cavity is different to the collagen present in the joints, so this is something to consider if you are looking into buying a collagen supplement.

Collagen supplements can come in different formats (powder, liquid, pills), which can impact their absorption into the body. In any case, when the collagen gets digested, it breaks down into amino acids in your stomach, so the collagen you put into your mouth becomes something different when it hits your stomach acids. Besides, collagen supplements have an animal or vegetable source, not human. The collagen of a cow may not be the same collagen that your prolapse needs.

To date, I haven't found any reliable research that reports improving prolapse symptoms by taking collagen supplements. In saying that, I have met people that reported experiencing an improvement in their prolapse symptoms when taking collagen and following a pelvic floor and core training program. More specific studies need to be done, but we know that exercise stimulates collagen synthesis,[39] and eating food rich in glycine and vitamin C could also boost collagen production.[40]

Regular physical activity, specific pelvic floor and core work, and eating food rich in collagen and glycine (such as bone broth or meat cuts close to the animal bone that have more tendinous tissue) and vitamin C can boost your collagen production without breaking the bank.

CORE TRAINING WHEN YOU HAVE A PROLAPSE

If you remember the response of the intra-abdominal pressure when performing a crunch exercise explained in the previous chapter. We can deduce that this type of exercise can also be detrimental to prolapse. So it's best to start with exercises that will restore the supportive capacity of your muscles and surrounding structures. As we covered earlier, pelvic support is linked to your posture and breathing, so focus on this first.

A prolapse needs to be taken seriously and requires a high level of care. If you commit to a holistic training program and the right habits, you will notice positive changes in your body, and your quality of life will improve. Refer to the exercise guide in the final chapter for a safe core training program for prolapse.

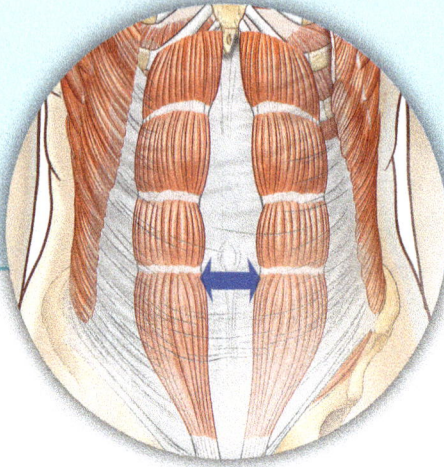

ABDOMINAL DIASTASIS:
TO CLOSE OR NOT TO CLOSE THE GAP

06

ABDOMINAL DIASTASIS: TO CLOSE OR NOT TO CLOSE THE GAP

YOU CAN HAVE A FUNCTIONAL CORE AND ABDOMINAL SEPARATION

ABDOMINAL DIASTASIS, a gap between the two sides of the rectus abdominis muscle (see the image below), seems to cause the most aesthetic concern for pregnant women. It naturally develops during the last stage of pregnancy because of hormonal changes in the mother's body and the expansion in the abdominal wall to allow for her baby's growth. It occurs when the two bands of the rectus abdominis separate because the collagen tissue that joins them (called the linea alba) stretches.

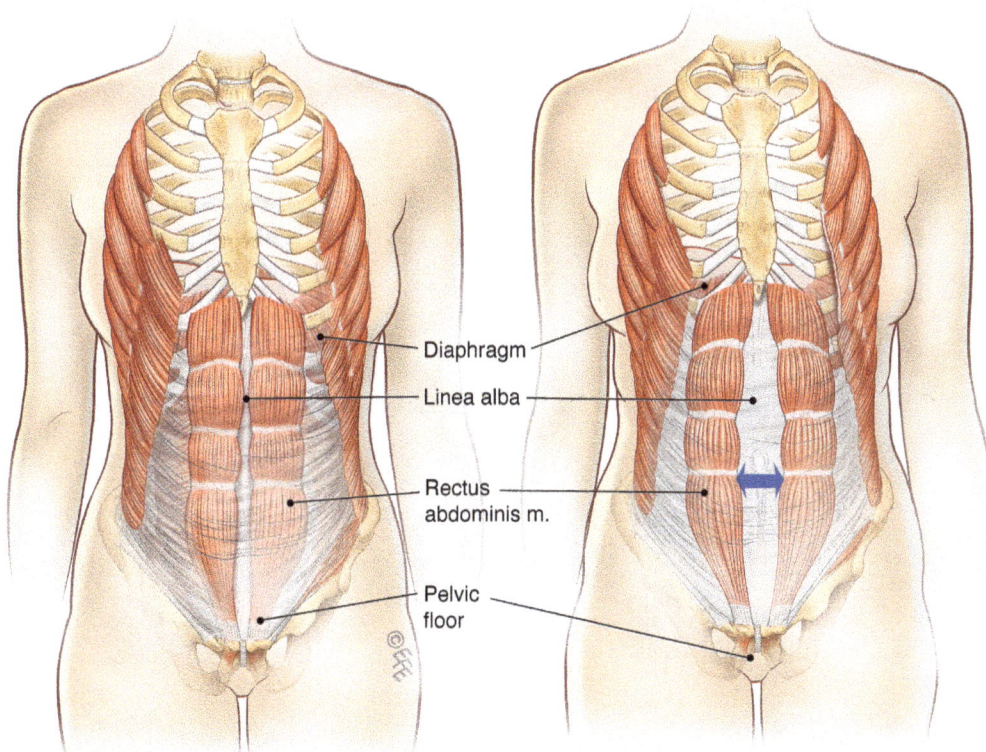

Diaphragm

Linea alba

Rectus abdominis m.

Pelvic floor

Diastasis is diagnosed when the tissue stretches beyond its natural limits. It is generally considered diastasis when there is more than 2cm of separation between the two abdominal bands. Diastasis can partially recover as part of the body's natural healing process after delivering a baby, particularly during the first weeks. But if nothing more is done, certain separation can remain permanent.

The "mummy tummy" is dreaded by most women aesthetically, but abdominal diastasis is more than that.

Although not the primary reason for back pain, the frightful gap can contribute to the development of lumbo-pelvic pain due to the instability of the abdominal wall and the lack of support.[41]

The doming observed in the belly when doing an abdominal curl shows the distortion of the tissues that have been overstretched and now remain unable to tense when the rectus abdominis contracts.

Current research indicates no clear relationship between abdominal diastasis and pelvic floor dysfunction.[42]

Interestingly, having diastasis doesn't make you more likely to have weaker pelvic floor muscles or more urinary incontinence or prolapse.[43] This can make us think that the stretching of the abdominal wall during the last months of pregnancy could be an adaptative mechanism of the body to protect the pelvic floor by dissipating the pressure in the pelvic cavity. On the other hand, a study on women with no pelvic floor dysfunction showed that deep abdominal muscle activation exists during pelvic floor exercises[44] which means the co-activation of these structures is important to guarantee the functionality of the core.

To date, there are no clear risk factors for diastasis. However, OBESITY, the number of pregnancies, MULTIPLE PREGNANCIES AND FLACCID ABDOMINAL MUSCLES can contribute to abdominal separation.[45]

HOW TO IDENTIFY IF YOU HAVE DIASTASIS

Ideally, diastasis should be assessed by a specialised health professional, i.e. a women's health physiotherapist, but if you are curious to find out if you have it, there's a simple way to feel for it.

Lay on your back with your legs bent, and lift your head and shoulders off the ground, curling your upper body up. While holding that position, gently press your fingers down the midline of your belly, starting at the top (close to your chest bone) and travelling down (until you reach your pubic bone).

Look for these things when assessing your diastasis:

- Separation between your two abdominal bands – how many fingers can you fit in the gap? It is commonly accepted that if you can fit more than two fingers, your separation is considered likely to be a problematic diastasis.

- The exact location of the separation (it's normally located around the belly button, but it can also happen above or below).

- The softness of the tissue in the gap: how far do your fingers sink in? If they sink too much into the diastasis, there is not enough tension in the midline tissues when the muscles contract which is a sign of a possible problematic diastasis. Feeling the tissue recoil can also give us an indication of the degree of damage on the linea alba.

WHAT CAN I DO ABOUT DIASTASIS?

When we talk about diastasis, there are two main aspects involved, one is aesthetical, and the other is functional. A closed gap does not necessarily mean the problem is fixed.

Working on the function of the core should be the priority.

You want to restore the capacity of the muscles and tissues to manage intra-abdominal pressure and be able to transfer the loads when performing your daily activities. If, after recovering the functionality, you still don't like how your abdominal wall looks, the solution may be in cosmetic surgery.

> **THERE IS LITTLE EVIDENCE AND KNOWLEDGE ON WHICH EXERCISES ARE MOST EFFECTIVE IN REDUCING ABDOMINAL SEPARATION.**

The main reason is the low methodological quality of the studies.[46] It has been commonly suggested that abdominal crunches should be avoided, and more gentle exercises such as abdominal drawing could be done. But these recommendations are based on best guesses, and, in many cases, abstaining from doing core exercises during pregnancy and postpartum is often the easiest solution offered by professionals, making the core potentially more dysfunctional and weaker.

In relation to whether doing crunches is good for diastasis or not, we have a couple of interesting studies. One of them has revealed the response of the linea alba and the gap measurement when performing different abdominal exercises. The study also shows that the slackness of the linea alba during an abdominal action is also a relevant aspect.

When we do a curl-up without activating the deep core (transversus abdominis), it will reduce the gap but can distort the tissues of the linea alba (this is evident in large diastasis when we see the doming in the belly when performing a crunch).

However, if we perform the same action activating the deep core may not reduce the gap distance but will generate a greater tension on the linea alba, which will increase abdominal support and optimise core function.[47]

Another study on pregnant and post-pregnant women compared the variations in the abdominal separation when doing an abdominal crunch and drawing in the abdominal wall.[48]

The results showed that:

- The drawing in exercise (pulling your belly in) generally leads to an *increase in the gap.*

- The abdominal crunch *significantly decreased the gap* compared to rest during the pregnancy and postpartum.

This comes to show that crunches can actually reduce the distance between abdominal bands and you can change the gap distance just by activating your core muscles differently during a curl-up movement.

> **DIASTASIS** is not just a problem of whether we should do crunches or not or whether we need to close the gap.

A holistic approach to diastasis healing can be more effective, considering most of us don't do any crunch-based movement patterns in our daily activities. Balancing the pressure in the core and correcting the posture and breathing will aid diastasis healing. Also, with all of your core muscles working in sync, good abdominal and pelvic floor tone, will be paramount for trunk stability and back and pelvic pain reduction.

In the following image, you can see an example of how good posture can contribute to diastasis correction by simply elongating the myofascial frontal chain of the body. Including exercises that promote spine elongation will help reduce the gap between the two abdominal bands.

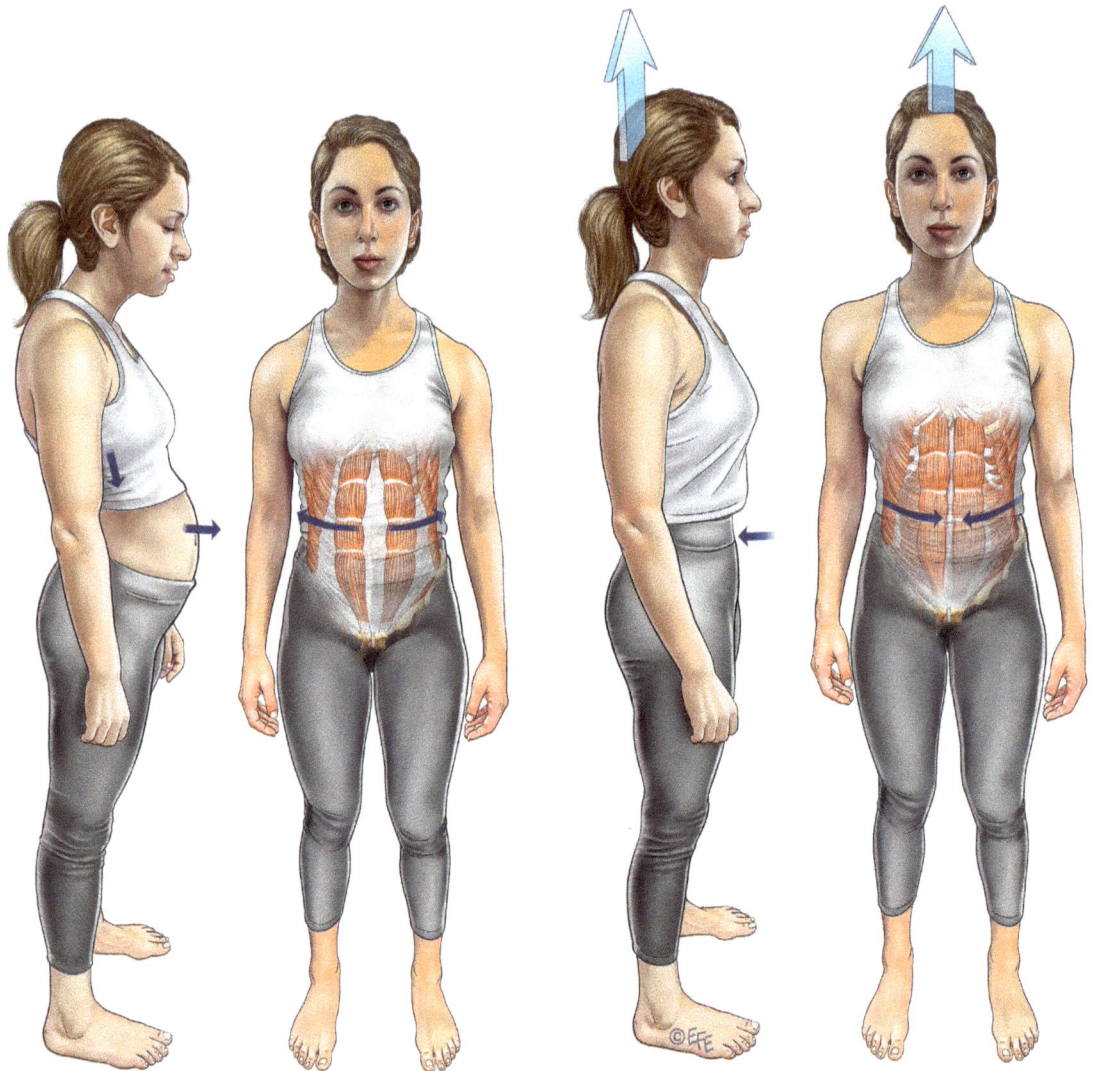

IS IT ONLY PREGNANCY THAT CAUSES DIASTASIS?

Abdominal diastasis is a problem affecting more than post-pregnant women; it can also be found in men, and young people. Excess intra-visceral fat can expand the abdominal wall the way a growing baby does during pregnancy. Men and women with overly large stomachs often suffer abdominal separation and should approach core training like pregnant women.

Have realistic expectations: Diastasis is normal in pregnancy, and the degree of separation depends on many factors, some of which have a genetic component, therefore, the healing process is different in every person and sometimes unpredictable.

A diastasis training program should focus on improving the strength and function of the abdominal wall from a holistic approach rather than just focusing on closing the gap.

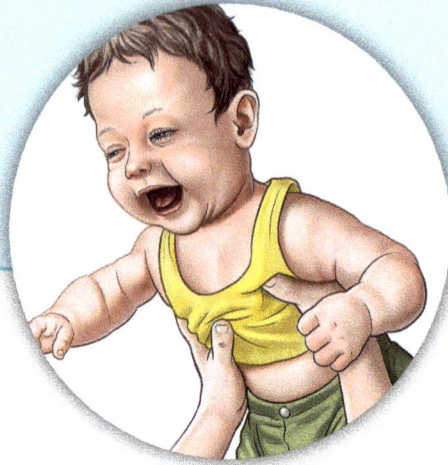

CHAPTER 07

POSTPARTUM:
A SAFE RETURN TO EXERCISE

07 POSTPARTUM: A SAFE RETURN TO EXERCISE

FORGET THE BOUNCE-BACK CULTURE AND THINK IN THE LONG TERM

Returning to exercise after giving birth is often confusing for new mums. Doctors recommend resting for six weeks after the baby is born, but what to do after is sometimes a big dilemma for women who are often desperate to get their pre-baby bodies back.

It's important to know that everyone is different; while some may be ready to start some form of exercise after six weeks, others may need more rest time or may need a specific program due to birth complications and/or fitness levels.

I recommend visiting a women's health specialist to assess the possibility of you getting back into exercise and recommending what type of exercise would be suitable.

TOO MUCH EXERCISE OR NOT AT ALL: FINDING THE RIGHT BALANCE

Incontinence, diastasis and prolapse are the number one enemies of post-natal women. When no one gives you the correct information about the changes in your body and how to exercise safely, you don't know what to do. Usually, one of the two extremes happens; you either try doing your pre-pregnancy exercise routine, or just stop doing any form of exercise.

Doing the right amount of the appropriate type of exercise adapted to your current fitness level is the right way to go.

Rushing into the same exercise routine you did before becoming pregnant will likely bring pain and dysfunction in the short and long term. Your body has undergone 42 weeks of significant physical and physiological changes; the muscles, ligaments and other tissues have stretched, and your internal organs have moved to make space for your growing baby. Also, the hormonal changes during pregnancy modify the composition of your connective tissue, making your ligaments and the muscles of your pelvic floor laxer in preparation for birth.

After nine months of changes in our body, we can't expect it to go back to normal in six weeks! After birth, the body undergoes more physiological and physical changes, and we need to RESPECT THE PROCESS.

Birth itself is more physically demanding than the hardest iron-man race, yet many women want to run a marathon only few months after giving birth!

This may be possible for some women, but not all. The process of recovering from childbirth requires patience and a gradual return to exercise that progresses at a different pace in different people.

On the flip side, some women decide not to exercise at all, which can be because they are scared of going back to exercises or hope their bodies will return to their pre-pregnancy state automatically. Although letting your body heal is probably better than doing the wrong thing at the gym, you do need to guide your body through the healing process.

Once you've had your baby, your body needs to prepare for the demands of having a child; lifting and holding the baby for extended periods of time, carrying the pram and putting it in the car, bending over to change nappies, that is a whole day's workout itself!

Doing the correct exercises to get your core, back, and pelvic floor working efficiently so they provide enough support should be your primary fitness goal six weeks after giving birth.

Doing nothing can lead you to the same problems you'd have if you were training too much – pain and dysfunction.

WHAT TO DO?

Firstly, visit your doctor to get clearance so that you can begin exercising gently. I also recommend seeing a pelvic floor specialist who can assess your muscles and internal organs and give you specific exercises for your body's recovery.

Secondly, be patient and listen to your body. It's best to return to exercise progressively, with the focus on restoring the function of your abdominal and pelvic muscles (they are the centre and most important part of your body). As covered in earlier chapters, it's not about making those muscles strong but rather ensuring they work in sync and according to the demands of your everyday physical activity.

Gravity works against your pelvic floor restoration and pelvic organ repositioning, so it's essential to avoid high-impact activities, heavy lifting, and standing for extended periods of time for the first 12 weeks at least. After that, you can progressively include these exercises into your routine as long as you maintain your core and pelvic floor function.

Parenting can be exhausting and finding one hour for yourself can be hard. Breaking your exercise down into small bursts throughout the day can make it more manageable than an entire one-hour session.

And lastly, if you are unsure about how to start exercising after birth, I recommend seeking a fitness professional with specialised training in pregnancy and postpartum who knows the needs and risks and will guide you in a safe return to physical activity.

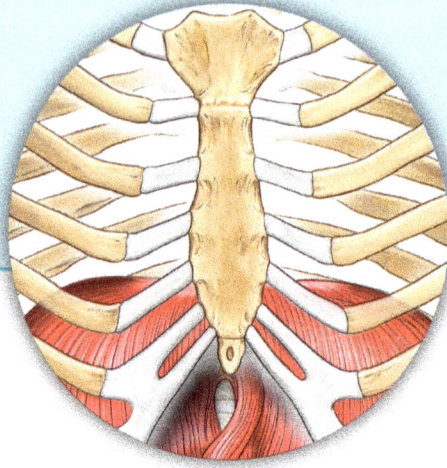

CHAPTER 08

A SPECIAL SECTION
FOR BLOKES

08 A SPECIAL SECTION FOR THE BLOKES

IT'S NOT ALL ABOUT THE SIZE OF YOUR BICEPS!

Many people think that men are free from the issues covered in this book because they don't give birth, but weakness in their core and pelvic floor muscles can also lead to different dysfunctions. The male abdominal wall and perineum are more supportive than females, thus protecting against increased abdominal pressure. However, their core still has its vulnerable points, and lifestyle and the type of exercise can also impact their core and pelvic floor health. Please invite the men you care about to read this chapter.

THE CORE ISSUES MEN FACE

INGUINAL HERNIAS

An inguinal hernia occurs when a weak spot in your abdominal muscles and some tissue – usually part of the intestine – protrudes. This is the most common hernia in males, with an estimated prevalence of 27–43% in males and 3–6% in females.[49] Although some hernias are congenital (present at birth), others develop over time.

When a pre-existing weak area in the abdominal wall is combined with repetitive actions that increase pressure, such as coughing, lifting, or any other strenuous activity, tissue can protrude out of the abdominal wall through the weak point.

Why are men more prone to inguinal hernia?

During male fetal development, testicles descend from the inside of the body through the abdominal lining into the inguinal canal. Usually, the abdominal lining closes over during the weeks after birth, but sometimes an opening is left that the intestine can slip through. This phenomenon is called an **Indirect Hernia.** Women also have an inguinal canal, which contains the ligaments that hold the uterus in place. Besides, the ovaries remain inside the body, making this area more supportive.

In contrast, **Direct Hernias** occur in older adults due to weakness in the abdominal wall, usually created by too much strain in the groin area because of strenuous activity or perhaps a persistent cough. They are typically found in athletes whose sports involve repetitive twisting and kicking, such as soccer, football, ice hockey, skiing, running and hurdling.[50]

Like pelvic organ prolapse, inguinal hernias can have differing degrees of complications. Initially, hernias do not necessarily cause symptoms, but if nothing is done and the hernia progresses, the contents of the abdominal cavity – such as the intestine or even the liver– can burst into the groin canal. This restricts the blood supply and causes obstruction, and surgery is needed to repair the tissues.

Signs of a possible hernia are:

- A bulge in the groin area on either side of your pubic bone
- The bulge becomes more noticeable when standing up, coughing or straining
- You experience pain or discomfort in the area
- There is heaviness or a feeling of pressure in the groin
- You experience pain when bending over, coughing or straining

CORE TRAINING AND INGUINAL HERNIA:

To prevent or manage inguinal hernia, be aware of your body, look for symptoms, and seek professional advice if you think you have one. A weak core increases the chance of suffering a groin hernia which is why maintaining the supportive capacity of your core muscles is essential to prevent it.

Inguinal hernias are negatively affected by increased pressure in the abdominal and pelvic cavity, so conventional core training exercises, impact activities and heavy lifting can cause further damage to the supportive structures and aggravate the condition. A gentle approach to exercise is needed.

DISC HERNIAS AND SLIPPED DISCS

Most of us know about disc hernias; they are common back injuries that can cause a lot of pain. But why do disc herniate? The intervertebral discs in your spine that sit between each vertebra are like small tyres made of cartilage and other fibrous tissues. On the inside of the tyre is a gel-like elastic substance that absorbs the impacts in the spine, allows movements without grinding the vertebrae, and protects the spinal cord. And just like with tyres, vertebral discs suffer wear and tear as we age, losing their water content and sometimes developing small cracks. A hernia occurs when the cartilaginous "tyre" tears and the gel inside is pushed out, where it presses on the spinal nerves and causes significant pain or numbness and weakness in the limbs.

What leads to disc herniation?

There are genetic factors that can predispose someone to have a disc hernia, but there are other external aspects that can increase the risk of disc herniation:

- Obesity increases the pressure on the spine and, therefore, on the intervertebral discs.[51]

- Repetitive movements that combine twisting and flexion of the spine.[52]

- Heavy lifting

- Sitting and driving for long periods

- Smoking, it's believed, speeds up the degenerative process of the vertebral discs.[51]

Disc hernias are slightly more common in males than females.[53] Preventive action is essential to reduce the chances of needing surgery. Maintaining your core function and your posture should be your primary fitness focus. Training your core to support your spine throughout your daily activities and sports will reduce the symptoms and the likelihood of surgery.

PROSTATE PROBLEMS

The prostate is a small gland, about the size of a walnut, located below the bladder and around the urethra. Its primary role is to produce the semen that protects and feeds the sperm cells. Enlarged prostate, prostatitis (inflammation of the prostate) and prostate cancer are three common prostate conditions in men. These conditions can impact bladder control and pelvic floor function, as the prostate rests on these muscles and has connective tissue and neural connections.

Excess abdominal fat will put pressure on the prostate and restrict blood flow in the area, as well as making it harder to support the internal organs. Maintaining a healthy weight is integral to prostate health and core function.

Just like the female's pelvic floor, physical activity that involves heavy lifting and impact will increase the pressure on the internal organs and the pelvic floor, including the prostate. If your prostate is enlarged or inflamed, this type of physical activity may not benefit these conditions. Sometimes prostate surgery is needed, leaving the muscles weak and causing urinary incontinence. The urinary sphincter is connected to the prostate by tissue and muscle fibres, which is why the removal of the prostate gland can lead to urine leakage. This can have a significant impact on men's quality of life.

Exercising the pelvic floor, in coordination with the core muscles and the diaphragm mobility, can offset the adverse effects of prostate surgery and optimise urinary function.[51]

ERECTILE DYSFUNCTION

Erectile dysfunction is the inability to achieve or maintain an erection. It is associated with other health and psychological issues, and getting the correct diagnosis of the underlying problem is essential. Although the role of the pelvic floor muscles in sexual function is often overlooked, there is a strong relationship between these muscles and having an orgasm. During sexual arousal, the blood flow concentrates in the penis thanks to the pelvic floor muscles helping to maintain the blood flow during erection and orgasm. When the muscles are dysfunctional, or too tight and therefore restrict the blood flow to the penis, it is difficult to reach and maintain an erection.

Appropriate pelvic floor training that helps maintain good muscle tone and control of these muscles will lead to better ejaculation control and intensification of orgasmic pleasure.

PUDENDAL NERVE ENTRAPMENT

The pudendal nerve is the main nerve of the perineum (the area between the anus and the scrotum). It branches out to innervate areas, including the anus, urethral and anal sphincters, pelvic muscles and the penis. Its primary role is to provide sensation to these areas and to maintain the tone of the pelvic floor muscles.

If this nerve gets compressed by the surrounding muscles, it can cause pain, numbness and dysfunction in the genitalia, rectum and urinary tract. Sitting for prolonged periods on a bicycle or practising sports that involve repetitive hip flexion can provoke the impingement of this nerve. The discomfort from pudendal nerve neuralgia can cause hypertonicity of the pelvic floor muscles. A physiotherapist specialising in the pelvic floor will be able to assess and diagnose pudendal nerve entrapment and provide the best treatment, which usually involves relaxing these muscles.

IN SUMMARY

Men can also suffer from pelvic floor and core dysfunctions due to bad posture, incorrect exercising and unhealthy lifestyles, which can significantly affect overall well–being. The pelvic floor is the foundation of the core (for both men and women), and taking care of it should be a priority.

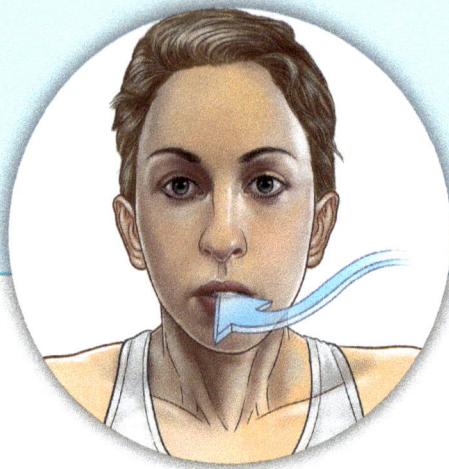

THE ESSENTIAL FIRST STEPS
TO TRAINING YOUR CORE

Visit paulacampanero.com to access the videos
of the exercises explained in this chapter.

09

THE ESSENTIAL FIRST STEPS TO TRAINING YOUR CORE

THE POWER OF BREATHING WELL

Doing the right exercises for your body – and particularly your core – is essential while still ensuring you enjoy it. A walk around the block for a sporty person experiencing core dysfunction won't be satisfying, so a program that includes exercises to improve core function and offsets the negative effects of your favourite sports is best. That way, you can keep doing the sports you love over the longer term.

EXERCISE IS VITAL whether you are a man or a woman, young or old, pregnant, trying to conceive or have just had a baby. A healthy fitness program should provide benefits and prevent pain or injury.

These final chapters are a practical guide to safely training and understanding your abdomen, pelvic floor, breathing and posture and will help you develop greater awareness of your body. The exercises I share are researched, effective alternatives to conventional core training.

If you are healthy and physically active, you can include the exercises into your regular fitness routine as a preventive measure. If you have a pelvic floor dysfunction, or a hernia or are recovering from birth, these exercises are a good way to help your body heal and prepare for future exercise.

If you are planning on getting pregnant, I strongly recommend you do them to ensure core function during pregnancy.

The exercises are a fusion of principles taken from different rehabilitation and exercise techniques such as myofascial release, postural and breathing re-education and hypopressive technique. They are very simple so can be practised daily, but if you are not that committed, do them at least twice a week. Besides, they do not require special equipment so you can practise them at home any time of the day.

LEARNING THE PRINCIPLES FIRST

Before diving into the exercises, we need to cover three simple steps that will set the foundation for a functional core. Do not underestimate the importance of these steps! They only take a few minutes and give so much insight into your body.

With the help of technology, you can record or photograph yourself while doing them; this can help you integrate what you see with what you feel and correct it as needed. Eventually, you will build your body awareness and be capable of feeling your own body movements and identifying correct performance without visual feedback. This is called proprioception.

1 RAISE BREATHING AWARENESS

Breathing patterns can affect core and pelvic floor function, so becoming aware of them and controlling and adapting them can be very useful.

Firstly, lie on your back and take a few deep breaths in and out, noticing which area of your body moves more: is it your shoulders and chest? Ribs? Abdominal area? You can place your hands on your chest, ribs and belly for different breaths to feel which part moves the most.

This exercise is best performed lying on your back so your abdominal wall is relaxed; however, you can do it in front of a mirror or record yourself breathing to have visual feedback.

If you notice that your chest and shoulders rise and tighten during inhalation, you are performing what is called shallow or chest breathing, which is how we tend to breathe when stressed (see image below).

Chest Breathing

Chest breathing mainly uses the muscles around our neck and chest to make room for the air coming into our lungs. These muscles can become tight and shorten over time which then causes the head to tilt forward, negatively affecting our breathing patterns.

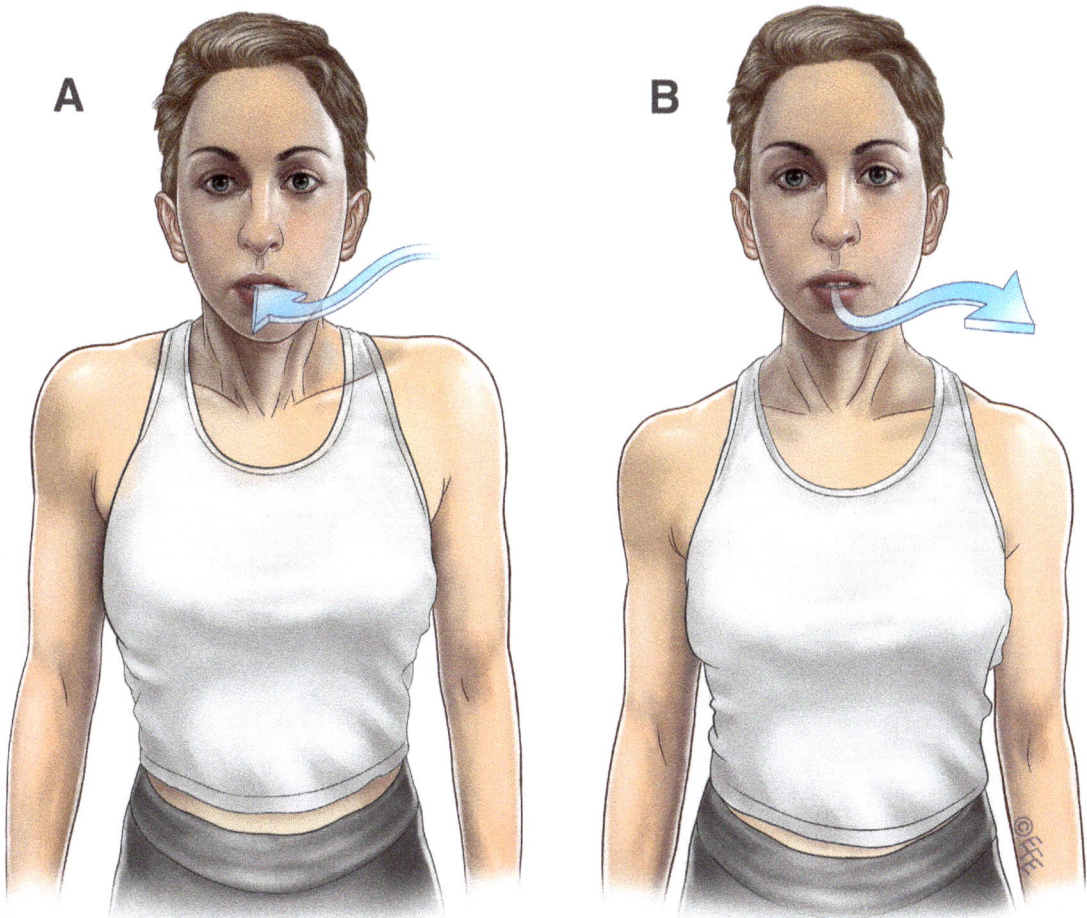

Abdominal Breathing

This is when you breathe with your belly. Place a hand over your belly button and feel how the abdominal wall expands as you inhale and how the belly relaxes and gently descends as you exhale. It is often taught as the best way to breathe to avoid shallow breathing. However, when your chest and the muscles around your ribs are too tight, the body will naturally find the path that offers the least resistance, the abdominal wall. Too much abdominal expansion can signal low muscle tone.

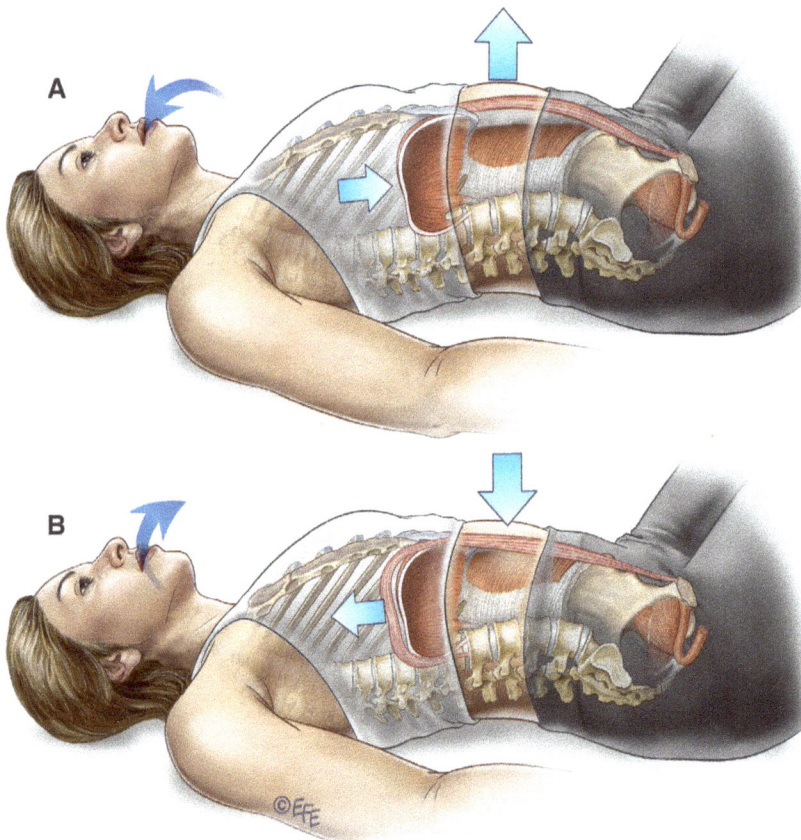

Additionally, expanding your belly does not necessarily mean that you are taking a deep breath in. Your abdominal muscles can expand without moving air pressure, so you may be expanding your belly, but your lungs are not actually filling. Your breath is still shallow, but you have shifted the pressure to your abdominal cavity.

Correct Diaphragmatic Breathing

This should be a combination of thoracic and abdominal movement – when you take a deep breath in, you should feel both your chest and your belly expand, and when you breathe out, you should feel both returning to their original position. During deep breathing, ribs move, not just your belly. Your lungs work the same way a balloon is blown up; they will expand in all directions when they have space.

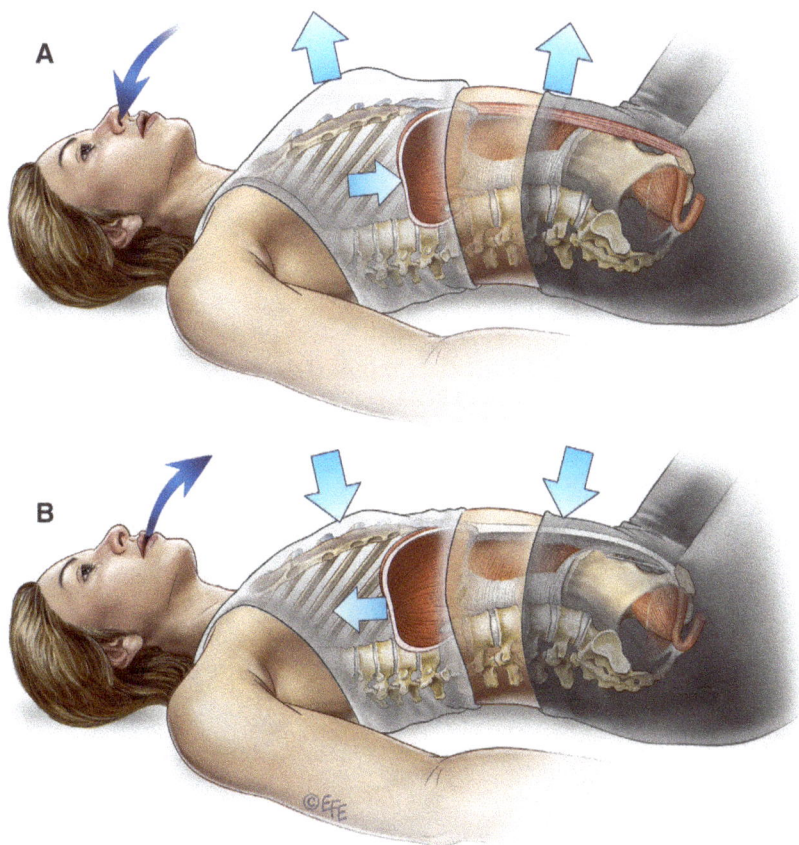

2 DISCOVER YOUR DIAPHRAGM

Correct movement of the diaphragm provides a number of health benefits. One of the best-known is the induction of relaxation to improve overall mental health and reduce stress.[55]

But it also has a positive impact on digestion, blood pressure and exercise performance, amongst many others.

The rib expansion produced during inhalation is often restricted because the diaphragm is tight, making it difficult to correct your breathing pattern. Luckily, you can do some simple exercises to release and mobilise the diaphragm and improve ribcage mobility.

EXERCISE 1: Massage the diaphragm to deepen the breath.

- Lie on your back with your legs bent and soles on the ground to completely relax your abdominal wall.

- Place your hands on the edge of your ribcage.

- Take a deep breath in, trying to expand your ribs as much as possible. Be careful not to tense your neck and shoulders.

- As you exhale, gently massage under your ribs with your fingertips. Pressing against them.

- Start massaging from the top, close to your chest bone and following down the line of your ribs on each breath.

- If you find a tender spot, stay in this region for a few breaths.

- Do this for at least ten breaths while keeping your abdominal wall relaxed throughout.

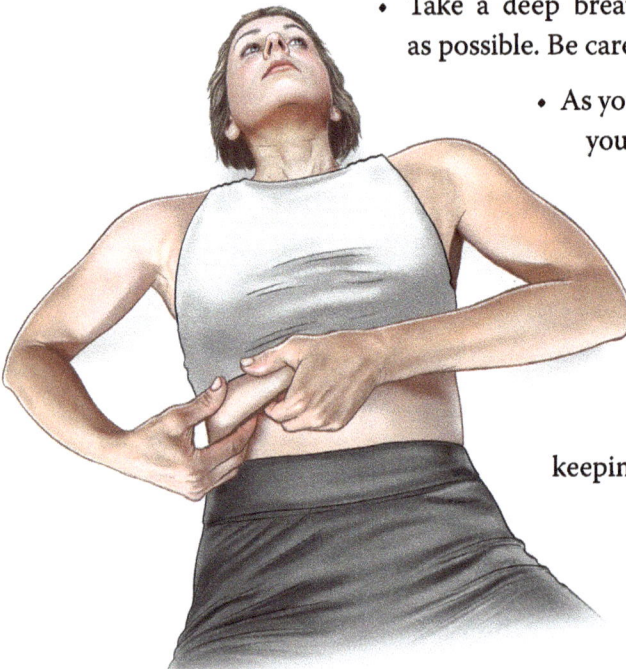

You don't have to massage too hard as the diaphragm reacts to slight pressure and is quite a sensitive area as well. While massaging, listen to your body and give yourself time. If you do this exercise regularly, you will notice the pain diminish and then disappear as the diaphragm relaxes.

EXERCISE 2: Mobilise your diaphragm and your ribs.

Once your diaphragm is less tense you can breathe into your ribs with more ease and perform this exercise better. Like Exercise 1, do this over a minimum of ten breaths.

- Lie on the floor with your legs bent and feet on the ground.

- Place an elastic band or something similar (a scarf or a thick belt) around your ribcage, crossing it at the front and holding each end with your hands. Maintain a certain level of tension in the band.

- Keeping your shoulders and neck relaxed, take a deep breath to feel how your ribs expand, pushing into the band.

- Exhale, letting the ribs return naturally back to the initial position.

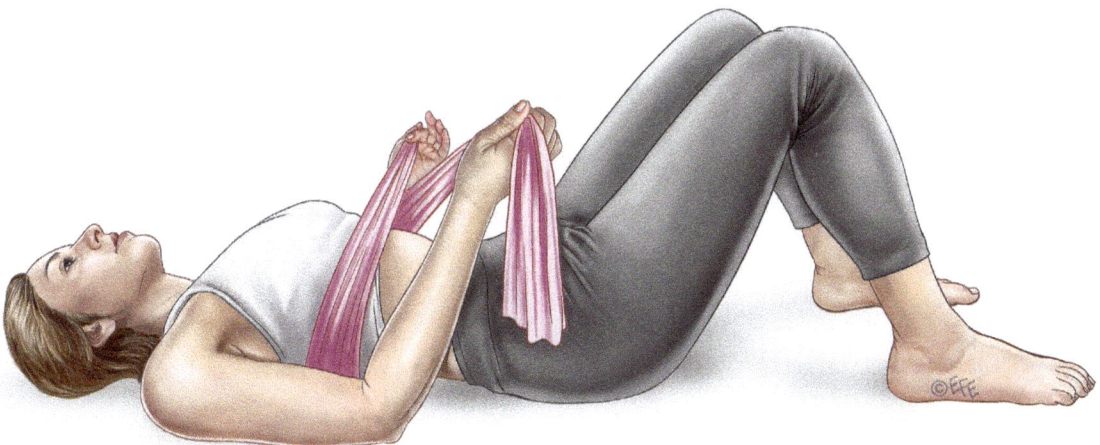

EXERCISE 3: Diaphragm-abdominal wall coordination

This exercise will help you visualize the correct movement pattern of your abdominal wall and diaphragm when breathing. Remember the breathing pattern explained in Chapter 4. Repeat this exercise for at least ten breaths.

- Lie on your back with your legs bent, feet on the ground, and hands holding the edge of your ribcage on each side.

- Take a deep breath in, expanding your ribs as much as possible without tensing the neck and the shoulders.

- As you exhale, hold your ribs to keep your ribs expanded. Don't let your ribs close during the exhalation.

- Feel how your abdominal wall descends as you exhale – you are now exercising your deep core muscles through breathing.

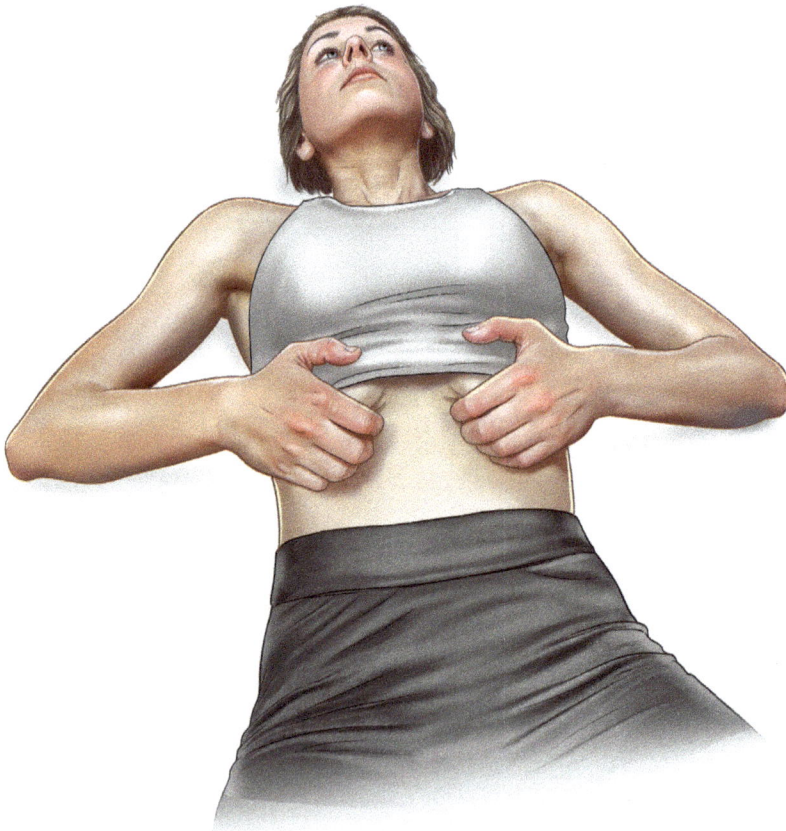

3 ASSESS YOUR POSTURE AND IDENTIFY THE CORRECT ALIGNMENT.

As previously mentioned, good posture is an important aspect of core health and function. Identifying proper body alignment will allow you to correct bad posture. To do this, you will need to take three full-body photos of yourself. So, you can observe your body, it is best to do it barefoot and wear fitted clothes.

1. Stand with your feet parallel hip-width apart, in your normal posture and looking ahead. Take a photo from the side.

2. Find an outer corner of a wall and stand with your back against it. Your heels, sacrum, shoulder blades and back of the head must be in contact with the wall. Take another photo from side.

3. In the same position, place a book on top of your head and feel as if you want to push into that book with the crown of your head, growing through the spine. Take another photo from the side while maintaining this position.

Once you have the three pictures taken, compare them looking for any differences. You will probably see that you look taller in the second and third pictures, but can you see anything else? Look closely at your abdominal area. Can you see that your belly looks slightly flatter in pictures two and three?

Good posture flattens your belly, thanks to myofascial traction. By simply elongating your spine, you can flatten your abdominal wall.

KEEP THE THREE PHOTOS on your records so that you can see the changes in your posture three months after following the exercises explained in this book.

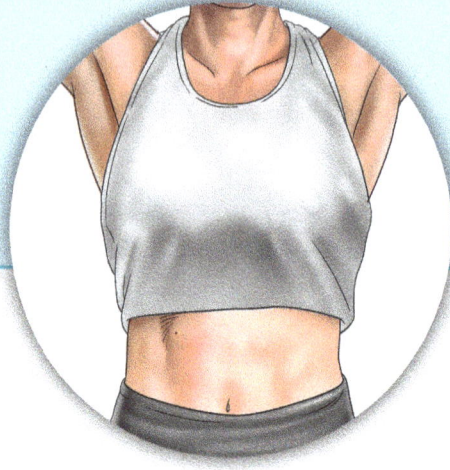

CHAPTER 10

HOW TO TRAIN YOUR CORE: THE EXERCISE SEQUENCE

Visit paulacampanero.com to access the videos
of the exercises explained in this chapter.

10

HOW TO TRAIN YOUR CORE: THE EXERCISE SEQUENCE

20 MINUTES A DAY IS ALL YOU NEED

Now it's time to integrate all the information in this book and transform it into actual exercises. The following sequence may look too simple or silly, but they are very effective if practised correctly. Please don't underestimate its powerfulness.

DIAPHRAGMATIC BREATHING PRACTICE

This exercise must be done at the beginning of your core training sequence. Begin by lying on your back with your legs bent and feet on the ground, though once you have more control, you aim to be able to do it in different positions such as sitting, on all fours and standing. This is what functionality is about.

As you learned in the previous chapter, diaphragmatic breathing involves a combination of rib and belly expansion. You have already practised the exercises that help improve and identify ribcage and diaphragm mobility. So now you better understand what needs to happen in order to breathe correctly.

WE DIVIDE THIS EXERCISE INTO THREE PARTS:

1 For at least three minutes, perform diaphragmatic breathing just focusing on what to do while inhaling: Breathe in through your nose (for the count of four) and fill your lungs, directing the air to your ribs first, expanding your ribs in 3D. Once you have reached full rib expansion, continue inhaling, directing the air to your belly. You can place one hand on your ribs and one on your belly to feel the movement. Exhale gently through your mouth (for the count of eight) with your lips and jaw relaxed as if you were fogging a glass.

2 For another 3 minutes, continue to breathe, but this time only focus on what to do while you exhale: Visualise the uplifting action that your pelvic floor and diaphragm to push the air out of the lungs as your abdominal wall slowly draws in. It's important to understand that it is not required to consciously activate the pelvic floor muscles in this action; however, an active visualisation of them performing the movement will help automate this pattern.

Imagine you are zipping up a pair of high-waisted 60s-style jeans. You start closing the zip on your pubic bone and continue up to your ribs. The action of drawing the belly in gently to close the zip is what we want to replicate here. This action finalises by letting the ribs return relaxed to the initial position without forcing them close, which could cause an unwanted downward pressure.

THIS IS THE BREATHING PATTERN YOU WILL MAINTAIN WHILE PERFORMING THE SEQUENCE OF EXERCISES I AM ABOUT TO EXPLAIN.

3 Now breathe, controlling your core movements while inhaling and exhaling. To keep it simple, inhale through the nose for the count of four and exhale through the mouth (fogging the glass) for the count of eight. This breathing pace can vary depending on how advanced you are in your practice and how comfortable you feel at that rhythm. Practise this for a minimum of three minutes as well.

When you have never been aware of how you breathe, this exercise can feel more difficult than you thought. Re-educating your breathing patterns requires patience and dedicated practice. Take your time to control your breathing in a lying position before coordinating it with the other poses.

THE EXERCISES SEQUENCE

The exercises may seem too simple to produce any effect on your body and your core, but they do. The secret is to maintain a slight activation of the muscles by keeping your spine aligned and activating your shoulder girdle (as explained in each exercise).

If you do the exercises with totally relaxed muscles, you will not achieve any results. Remember that maintaining the activation of the muscles is how we improve their tone through stimulating the slow twitch fibres of our postural muscles.

By correcting our posture with these poses we are ensuring that the pressure on the core walls is well managed and equally distributed on all surfaces. It is also important to make the breathing pattern while doing the exercises as it is effectively your "core work".

The goal is that during the 10 to 20 minutes you are performing the exercise sequence, you are constantly focused on your ELONGATED SPINE, ACTIVATED SHOULDER GIRDLE, CORRECT ALIGNMENT and BREATHING.

The sequence comprises four simple poses you will hold for at least ten diaphragmatic breaths before moving on to the next pose.

STANDING UP:

For beginners, perform this exercise with your back against the wall for constant feedback on your spinal alignment. You will also need an elastic band, scarf or belt.

- Stand with your feet parallel, hip-width apart, and with your heels in contact with the wall.

- Soften your knees, so they are slightly bent

- Make sure your sacrum, shoulder blades and the base of your skull are in contact with the wall and maintain the natural curves of your spine (as shown in the illustration).

- Position your head so your eye line is straight ahead and your chin neutral.

- Elongate your spine, pushing up towards the crown of your head as if you are growing taller. You can place a book on top of your head to remind you of this action. It is important to maintain spinal elongation the entire time as it activates the tonic muscles responsible for your posture. If you just stand up against the wall, you will not activate those muscles, and the exercise will be ineffective.

- Now position your arms as shown in the image, holding the band with your hands between your thumb and palm (see image).

- Broaden your chest without squeezing your shoulder blades to-gether; instead. make them feel like they are spreading outwards to the sides.

- Maintaining a slight tension on the band with your hands, gently drop your shoulders down as if you wanted to put your shoulder blades into your butt pockets and reach your arms down with your fingertips while maintaining contact with the wall.

- Slightly move your arms back, so you are pulling the band against your thighs. Feel this action is created by your muscles around your shoulder blades and not around your neck. Don't create too much tension on the band, just enough to maintain it through ten breathing cycles.

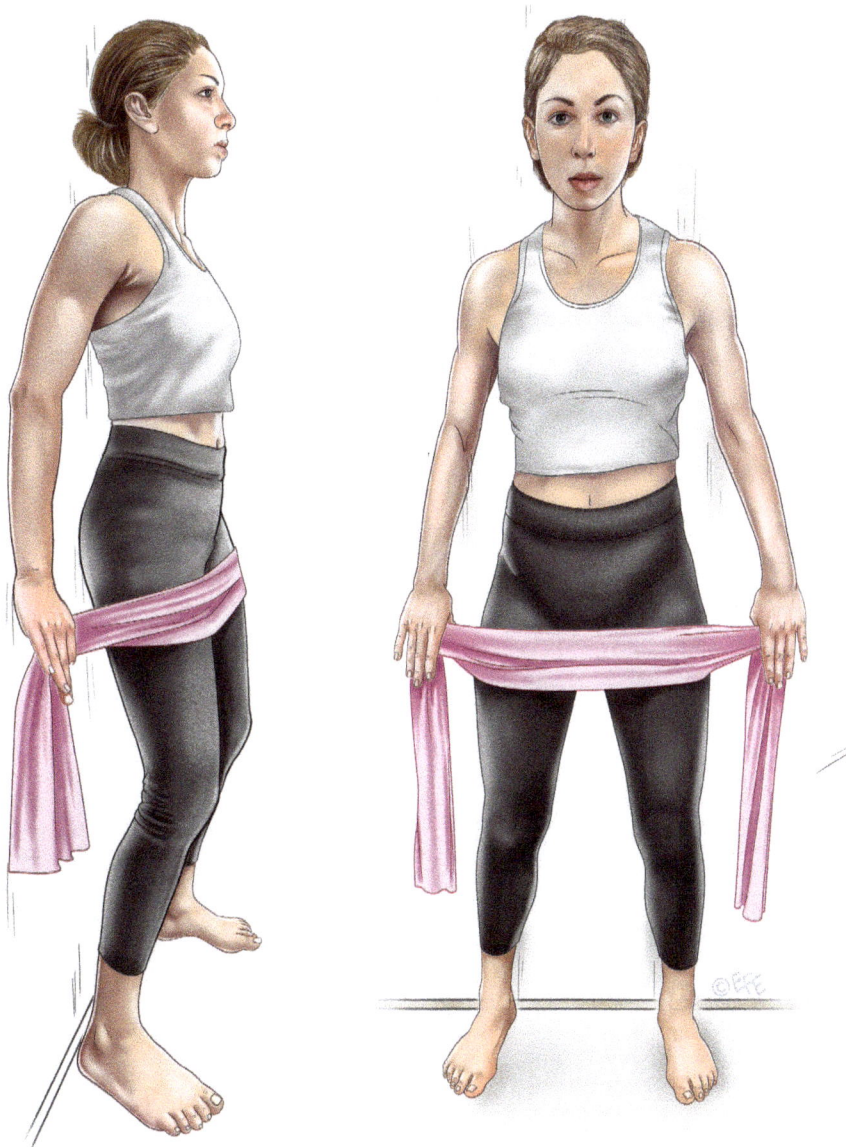

Hold this position as you perform at least ten diaphragmatic breaths and focus on the slight muscle activation caused by the maintained elongation of the spine and arms. Imagine your neck getting longer with each breath and your ears moving upwards and away from your shoulders.

PROGRESSION

Once you have gained more body awareness, you will be able to progress into the exercise without the different props slowly:

1. **Elongate the spine without having a book on your head.**

2. **Maintain spinal alignment without standing against the wall.**

3. **Activating your shoulder girdle and elongating your arms without holding an elastic band.**

VARIATION

You can perform this pose with your arms reaching up and partly to the sides.

In this position, the object is to elongate your arms without raising your shoulders. Reaching away through your fingertips

Just as in the first exercise, you can perform it first against the wall, feeling the contact of your arms and flat shoulder blades, and once you have gained body awareness in that position, move away from the wall.

The position of the arms above the head facilitates rib expansion and stretches the myofascial chain from the fingertips to your chest muscles. This chain tends to become tight due to daily activities involving the "closure" of the arms and hands. These include nursing a baby, carrying shopping bags, holding tools etc.

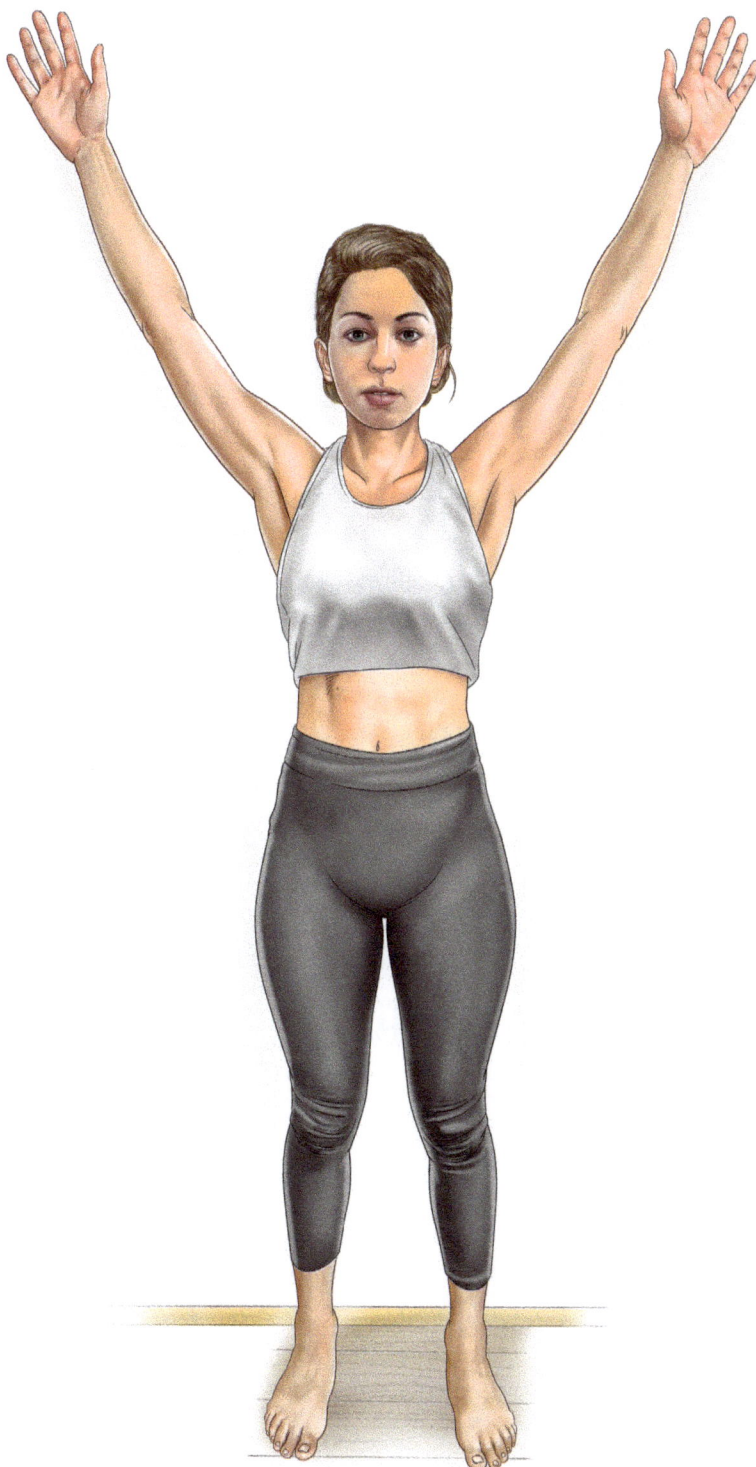

AGAINST THE WALL:

This time, stand facing the wall. Approximately half a meter away from the wall. With your feet parallel hip-width apart, and knees slightly bent.

- Your pelvis and spine are in a neutral position, maintaining elongation through the spine.

- Lean forward, so your hands meet the wall. Your body will be slightly inclined, with the weight held by your arms. Make sure your whole body is in a straight line, and you are not bending through the pelvis.

- With your hands placed shoulder width apart on the wall, rotate your arms so your fingertips face each other. And slightly bend your elbows, forming a round shape with your arms as if you were hugging a tree.

- Activate the shoulder girdle by pulling your shoulders down and spreading the shoulder blades out. As if you were pushing a wall with your elbows.

- Your head and chin are in a neutral position, and your eye line is straight to the wall.

- Maintaining this position, perform diaphragmatic breathing.

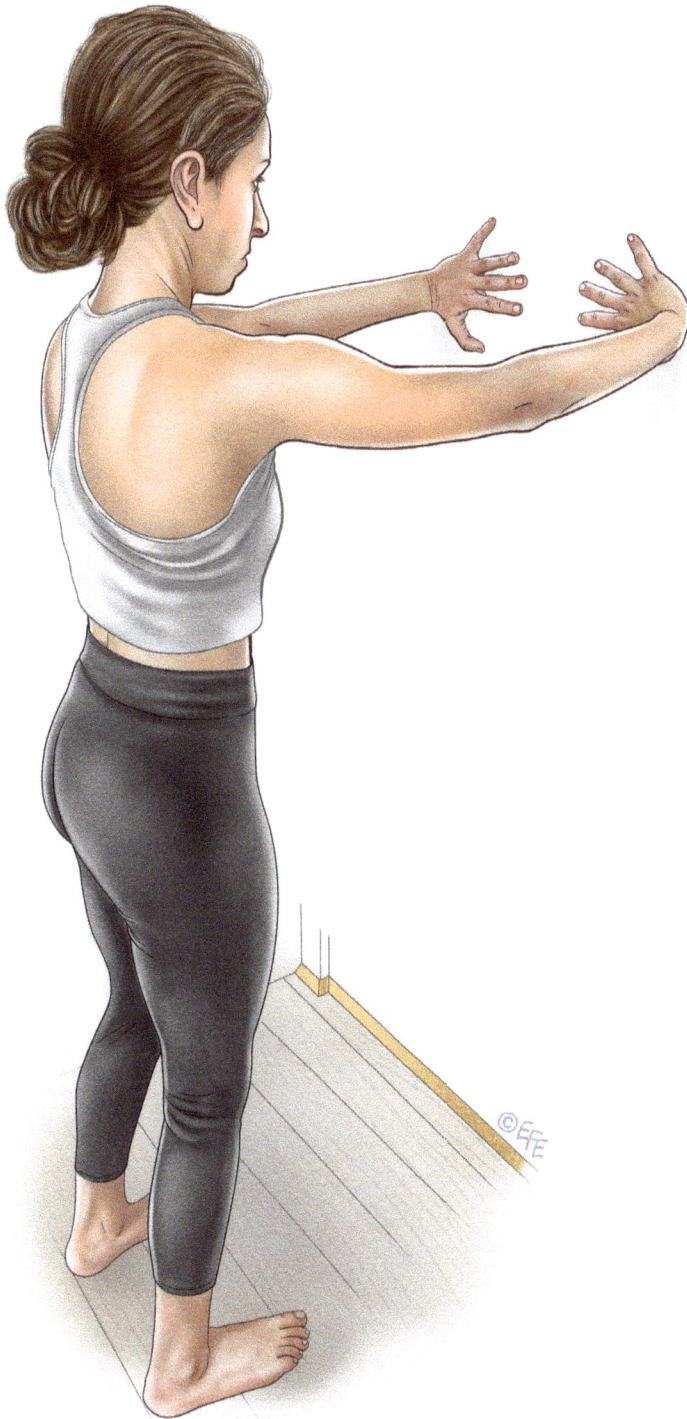

HIP HINGE:

In this pose, you need to stand in front of a table, approximately half a meter away from it and with your feet parallel, hip-width apart.

- Hinge through the pelvis, placing your hands on the table and bending your knees slightly. Keep your back straight and your head in alignment with the spine. Elongate from the tailbone to the crown of the head.

- With your hands on the table, shoulder width apart, internally rotate your arms so your fingers face each other. Bend your elbows slightly and make sure your chest stays broad.

- With your arms in that position, activate the shoulder girdle by slightly pushing with your hands into the table, with your elbows out (as if you were pushing walls) and with shoulders down.

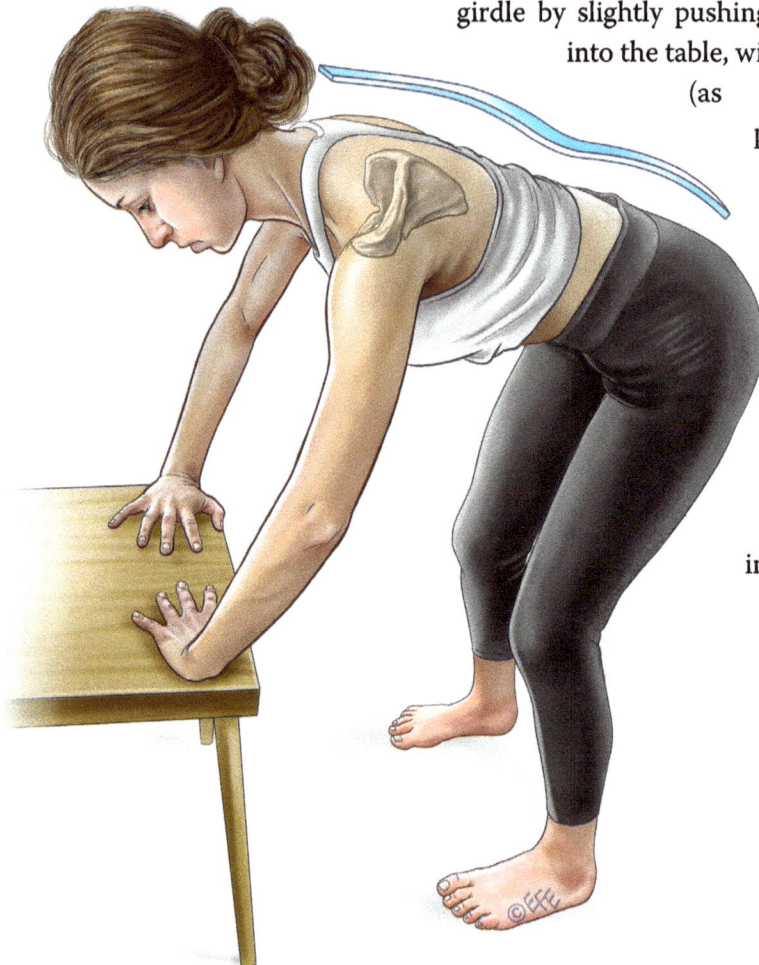

- Once in that position, maintaining the muscle activation and elongation, perform the breathing.

VARIATION

Once you master this pose, you can progress into a free-standing pose.

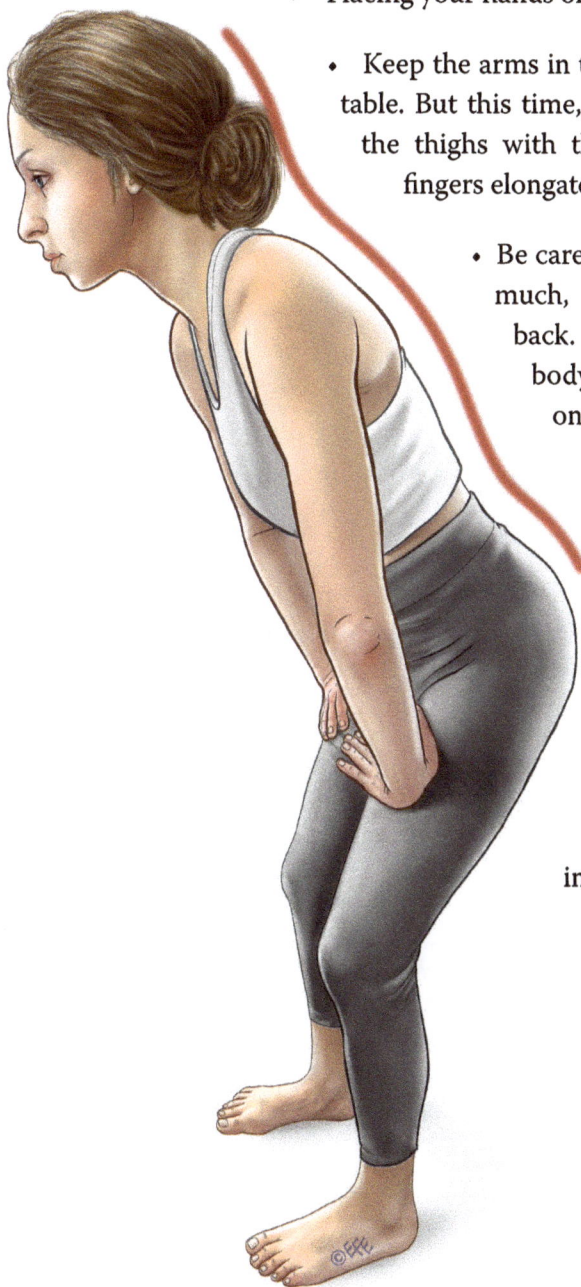

- Placing your hands on your thighs, close to your hips.

- Keep the arms in the same position as they were on the table. But this time, your hands are slightly pressing into the thighs with the heel of the hands, keeping your fingers elongated, not relaxed.

- Be careful not to incline your upper body too much, as that would overload your lower back. The level of inclination of your upper body is similar to the action of going to sit on a chair.

- Keep your spine straight maintaining its natural curves and elongating from the tailbone to the crown of the head.

- Activate your shoulder girdle in the same way as previously described. Pull the shoulders down, broaden your chest, and push with the elbows out and your hands into your thighs.

ON ALL FOURS:

For this exercise, you need to kneel on the floor in the same way as the image below.

- Place your elbow directly under your shoulders, with your forearms stretching forward and parallel to each other.

- Place your knees directly under your hips. Keep your feet in dorsiflexion and your heels in alignment with the legs (don't drop them to the sides). If you have pain in your ankles or toes holding that position, place a rolled towel under your ankles to release weight from the joints.

- Keep your shoulder blades flat; you mustn't sink into your shoulder blade.

- Place your head in alignment with the spine. If you place a bar along your spine, your sacrum, shoulder blades area, and back of your head should be touching it as the line represented in the image.

- Your eyeline is pointing to the ground, in between your forearms. That will help keep your head in the correct alignment.

- Activate your muscles by elongating your neck and pulling the shoulders back. Visualise your spine being pulled from your tailbone and the crown of your head.

- Maintain this position as you perform ten diaphragmatic breathing cycles. Feel how your ribs and abdominal wall expand as you breathe in and how they draw in and up as you exhale. Make sure you are not bracing your abdominals in this exercise.

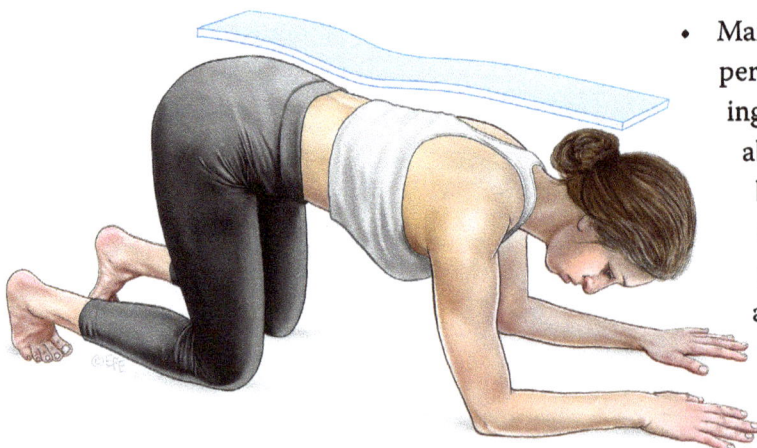

VARIATION

This is often the favourite pose for those who suffer from prolapse, as the inverted position helps reduce pressure on the abdominal cavity, enhances the uplifting action during the exhalation phase and reduces the chances of pushing out towards the pelvic floor.

- Slide your elbows out until your forehead can touch the ground as your hands move closer. You are forming a triangle with your elbows and your hands. And your head rests below your hands.

- Keep your shoulder blades flat and stable. Your body weight must be supported by your shoulders, not your head and neck. You should be able to move your head with ease in this position.

- Maintain the alignment of your spine as represented in the illustration.

- Activate your muscles by pulling your shoulders back and gently pressing your forearms into the floor.

- Spread your shoulder blades by pushing out with your elbows.

- Maintain this position as you perform the ten **breathing cycles.**

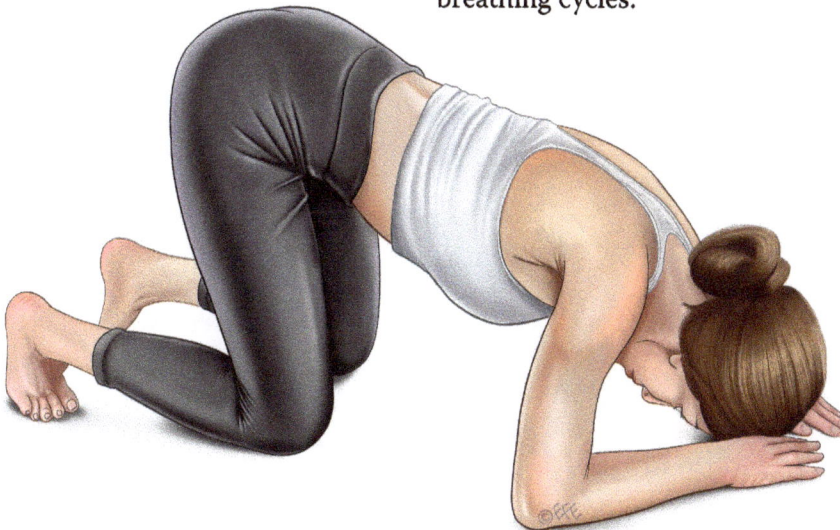

SITTING:

Sit with your legs crossed and your back against the wall. If it's uncomfortable for you, sit on an elevated surface such as a block or a cushion that will help you to sit upright., You can uncross your legs and have them bent slightly forward if you have issues with your knees. If you cannot sit on the floor at all, you can sit on a chair.

- Elongate your spine by placing a book on top of your head and pressing your head upwards towards the book.

- Place your arms onto your knees in the same way the image shows and activate your upper back by gently pressing your arms into your knees and pushing away through the heel of your hands.

- Make sure your chest is broad while having your arms in this position. Remember to maintain your shoulder blades flat against the wall. That will stop your shoulders from rolling forward.

- Drop your shoulders down and away from your ears and elongate your neck.

- Maintain the alignment and the shoulder activation, as you perform ten diaphragmatic breathing cycles. Know that in this position, you may find it harder to perform rib expansion, which is normal; just keep working on it, and it will become easier with practise.

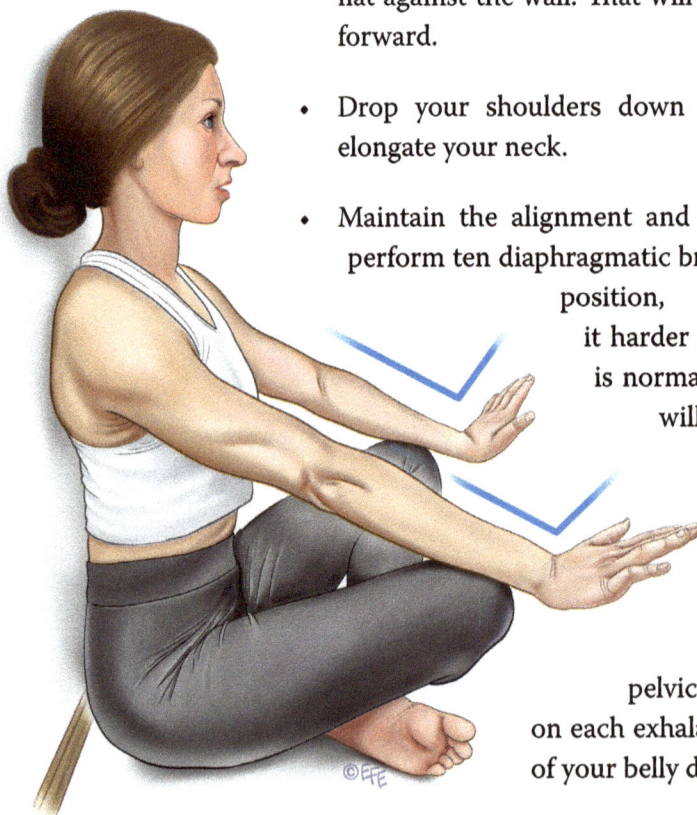

  - Every time you exhale don't "deflate" your body; instead, visualise the air being expelled from your body as if it came from your pelvic floor, and lengthen your spine on each exhalation. Feel the natural movement of your belly drawing in as you breathe out.

As you gain body awareness, progress into this exercise by moving away from the wall to maintain spine alignment.

VARIATION

Sitting in the same position with your arms reaching up and to the sides, like in the standing pose. First against the wall, then away from it. Maintain the chest broad and the shoulders down as the arms are reaching out.

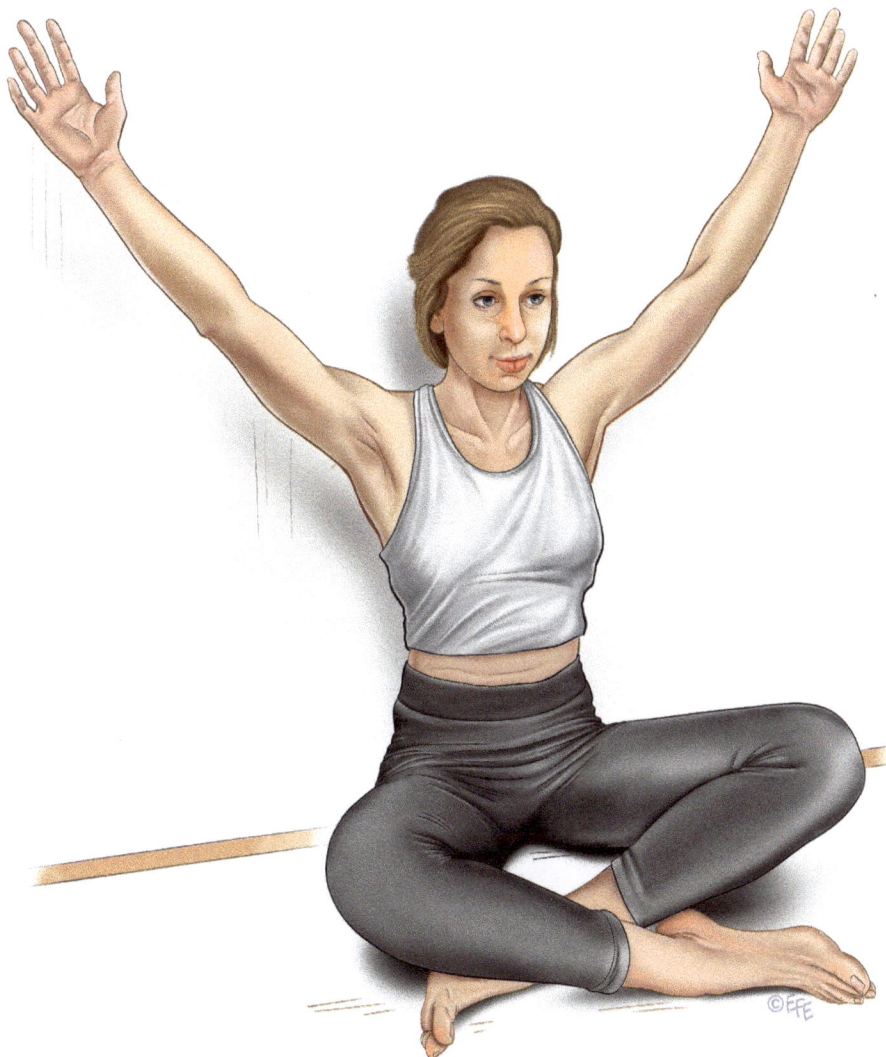

LAYING DOWN:

Lie on your back as shown in the image, with your feet flat on the wall and your knees at a ninety degrees angle.

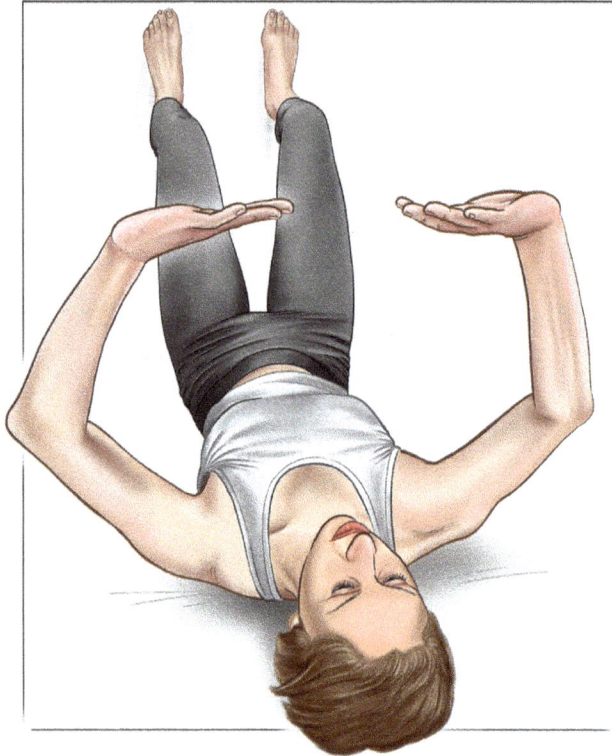

- Lift your arms to the ceiling, shoulders width apart, with your fingers pointing at each other, and in that position, slightly bend your elbows. Forming a circle with your arms as if you were holding a big ball.

- To activate your muscles, elongate your spine through the crown of the head. Make sure your chin is neutral and your eye line is to the ceiling.

- Pull the shoulders down and visualise as if you were pushing two walls with your elbows and, at the same time, pushing into the ceiling with the palms of your hands.

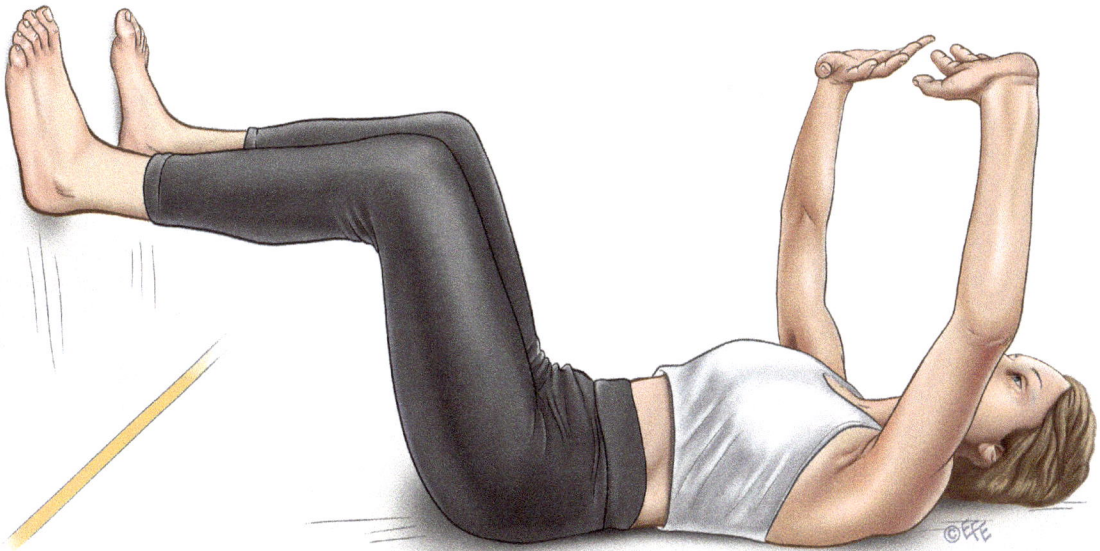

- Press slightly with your feet into the wall to activate your leg muscles.

- Maintaining the muscle activation in that position, perform the ten breathing cycles.

STRETCHING OUT:

This pose is designed to act upon the frontal crossed myofascial chains. Although it is easy and relaxing, it's important to maintain muscle activation, as described below.

- Lie on your back, as shown in the image. Make sure you cross your right ankle over your left and your feet are in the midline of your body.

- Place your arms above your head at an angle that allows you to maintain the natural curves of your spine. Do not arch your back trying to reach the ground with your hands. The range of motion you can do with this action depends on your shoulder flexibility.

- Your left hand is on top of the right, with the palms facing out and your elbows slightly bent, forming a circle with your arms.

- Activate your muscles by flexing your ankles and pushing away through the heels as if you were elongating and stretching your legs out of your hips.

- Pull your shoulders down and reach the crown of the head towards your hands, creating neck elongation.

- With your elbows slightly bent, push them out to the side into imaginary walls.

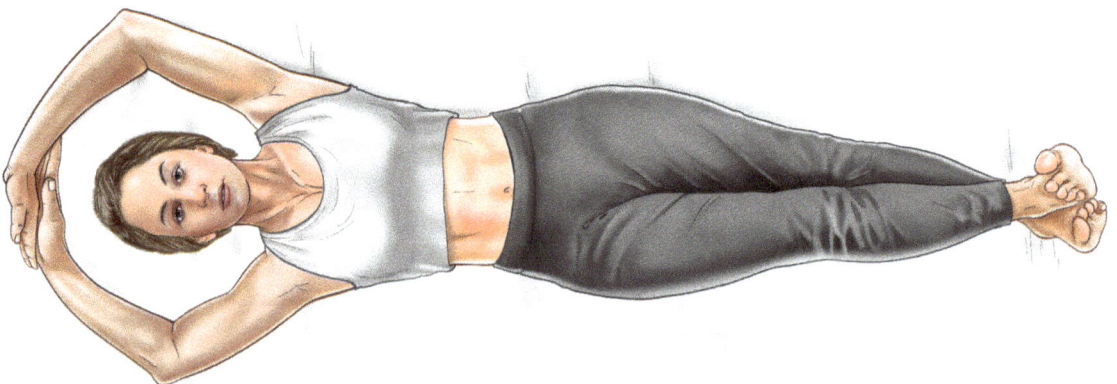

- Push your hands up and away from your body as if they were pushing into a wall.

- Maintain this muscle activation for ten diaphragmatic breaths, then switch your legs and hands and repeat for another ten.

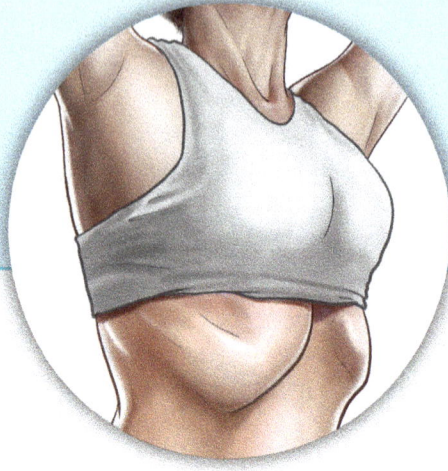

ENHANCE YOUR CORE FUNCTION WITH THE HYPOPRESSIVE TECHNIQUE

Visit paulacampanero.com to access the videos
of the exercises explained in this chapter.

11

ENHANCE YOUR CORE FUNCTION WITH THE HYPOPRESSIVE TECHNIQUE

THE EVOLUTION IN CORE TRAINING

If you want to take your core training to the next level, you can have a go at hypopressive training. The hypopressive breathing technique enhances the benefits for your pelvic floor and core by creating an intense inner stretch in your abdominal area and diaphragm.

WHAT IS THE HYPOPRESSIVE TECHNIQUE?

This technique was created in the 1980s by Marcel Caufriez, a Belgium doctor specialising in Women's Health. It was initially developed for treating pelvic floor dysfunctions and post-partum recovery, but soon became a preventive form of exercise for men and women.

The practice of HYPOPRESSIVES is widespread throughout America and much of Europe today. Athletes and bodybuilders use it as a TRAINING TOOL to prevent injuries and enhance specific training strategies.[56,57]

The word 'hypopressive' is a combination of the prefix hypo, which means low, and the word pressure. Thus 'hypopressive' means low pressure, which describes the main characteristic of this technique – to reduce intra-abdominal pressure. This is achieved by doing a series of postural and breathing exercises. Part of this technique has been explained in the previous chapter with the exercises and diaphragmatic breathing, but during hypopressive training, this planned sequence of poses is performed alternating diaphragmatic breathing with what we refer to as ABDOMINAL VACUUMS.

The abdominal vacuum is similar to an ancient yoga practice called *Uddiyana Bhanda,* in which the breath is held after a deep exhalation, and a controlled rib expansion is performed.

During this action, the core is elongated upwards, the diaphragm acts like a plunger. This produces a vacuum effect on the abdominal area, pulling the abdomen in and the internal organs and tissues upwards.

This anatomical response stimulates a natural co-activation of the core walls that will become automatic with regular practice.

ENGAGE THE DEEP ABDOMINAL MUSCLES WITH CONSCIOUS COORDINATION OF THE DIAPHRAGM.[58]

As discussed earlier in this book, the increase of IAP produced by our daily activities can be detrimental to our core and pelvic floor function. The hypopressive technique helps offset the negative effects of these actions and maintains the functionality of this group of muscles.

There is a common misconception that hypopressive training improves pelvic floor and core strength, leading to inaccurate research that compares the effects on pelvic floor muscle training and hypopressive training in muscle strength.

It is important to understand that hypopressive training is a holistic approach that aims to improve overall posture and breathing patterns and optimize core and pelvic floor function.

The benefits are way broader than just being able to contract your pelvic floor or your transversus abdominis. Hypopressive training is NOT an alternative to Kegels. It is a complementary training tool.

THE HYPOPRESSIVE TRAINING SYSTEM IS A COMBINATION OF THE FOLLOWING COMPONENTS:

Postural Techniques

As we have seen in previous chapters, posture impacts overall core function.

Breathing Techniques

Diaphragmatic breathing that we have already seen and the abdominal vacuum we will see in this chapter.

Myofascial Stretching

To normalise muscular and fascial tension in the body

Neurodynamics Techniques

To reduce neural tension and improve the function of the nervous system to adapt to mechanical loads and different movements.

Neuroeducation

Also known as brain-based education. The processes that take place in the brain during the learning process. The way the hypopressive training is taught will have an impact on the person who is learning.

After considering all these aspects we can see how hypopressive training can provide a wide range of benefits, even if you don't have pelvic floor or core dysfunction.

Incorporating this technique into your regular training routine will not only help you prevent them, but also help improve your overall health. Below you can read some of the benefits that have been proven by research:

PELVIC ORGAN PROLAPSE

One of the most common uses of hypopressive training is treating pelvic organ prolapse symptoms. The different poses are designed to improve overall posture and reduce pressure in the abdominal cavity.

When performing the abdominal vacuum, we create a shift that reduces intra-abdominal pressure in the pelvic cavity. At the same time, the plunger effect the diaphragm makes during this action also generates an internal lift of the pelvic organs[59] that helps to reposition them.

The regular repetition of this action will stimulate the tissues and the muscles to become more supportive and reduce the pain and heaviness so common in this condition.

PELVIC FLOOR MUSCLES, INCONTINENCE AND POST-PARTUM REHABILITATION

Although hypopressive training is not aimed at improving pelvic floor muscular strength, regular practice can help improve the ability to identify and properly contract the pelvic floor muscles and other muscles involved in pelvic and core stability, which in turn will have a positive impact on the treatment of stress urinary incontinence.[60–62] This is explained by the reflex activation of the muscles generated while maintaining the poses and performing the diaphragmatic breathing and abdominal vacuum.

This activation can be maintained for over ten seconds. Although it is not at an intensity high enough to induce muscle hypertrophy (muscle mass growth) and strength development, it is enough to improve muscle endurance.

If you remember from chapter three, muscle endurance is regulated by slow muscle fibres that can maintain a low-intensity contraction for extended periods of time, and this capacity regulates posture and continence.

CORE STABILITY AND POST-PARTUM REHABILITATION

A small study has found that when performing the yoga technique Uddiyanda Bhanda, there is an activation of the deep abdominal muscles as well as the pelvic floor.[63] Given this yoga practice is performed in a similar way to the hypopressive abdominal vacuum, we can extrapolate these findings to the hypopressive technique. Other researchers conducted studies specifically done with hypopressive training to prove this hypothesis.

The results have shown activation of the deep core and suggest that the hypopressive technique can be a good alternative to traditional core training without overloading the pelvic floor muscles by preventing an increase of downward pressure in the abdominal and pelvic cavity.[64,65]

This also means it can be safely used in post-partum rehabilitation along with other therapies and training.

MALE PELVIC FLOOR – PROSTATECTOMY RECOVERY:

As we already know, men also have pelvic floor muscles that weaken. Prostatectomy is a standard procedure in treating prostate cancer, but this procedure often results in urinary incontinence, which affects men's quality of life in many ways (socially, sexually and physically). Several studies have included hypopressive exercises in the treatment of urinary incontinence after prostatectomy with positive outcomes. [66–68]

This relies upon the fact that pelvic floor muscles have a much better activation when the surrounding abdominal muscles contract at the same time. Something that we have just seen occurring during hypopressive training.

In addition, optimising the breathing patterns by improving the co-ordination of the diaphragm with the abdominal and pelvic floor muscles can help reduce stress urinary incontinence.[20]

DIASTASIS

We have spoken about abdominal separation in chapter seven and know, at this point, there is not enough evidence to design the "perfect and only" protocol to treat abdominal separation. But based on the latest findings, we know that it is not all about closing the gap and other factors, such as connective tissue and muscle response when activating the abdominal wall, plays a big role in the equation.

A small study has been done on post-partum women with abdominal separation. After a four-week training program performing hypopressives, they experienced a reduction of abdominal separation and an improvement of the properties of the surrounding tissues and muscles.

These changes remained for up to two months after finalising the training program, which suggests that hypopressive training can be a safe and useful tool for core work when diastasis exists. However, it is also suggested that further studies with different procedure designs should be performed to achieve conclusive findings about the efficacy of this method in the treatment of diastasis.[69]

Other small studies have been performed with similar findings concluding that hypopressive training can be used in diastasis restoration and can be incorporated into post-partum recovery. However, further research is needed with a larger population, and the treatment for diastasis may need to be personalised and adapted to each case.[70,71]

BACK PAIN AND POSTURE:

The poses included in abdominal hypopressive training are designed to normalise overall myofascial tensions along with the diaphragmatic breathing and abdominal vacuum that reduces tension in the internal tissues and diaphragm attachments. All these effects seem to positively impact the treatment of lower back pain by improving the mobility of the back muscles and enhancing core muscle activation.[72]
Additionally, combining the abdominal vacuum with the postural

techniques induces activation of tonic muscle fibres (slow twitch fibres), which should increase the synergistic activation of all postural muscles and thus, improve posture control.[73]

CONSTIPATION

Constipation can harm pelvic floor health. Constant straining can weaken the pelvic floor muscles and put a lot of stress on the pelvic organs, aggravating prolapse symptoms. It can also negatively impact continence as the rectum and the bladder are very close in the pelvic cavity. If the rectum is full due to constipation, it puts excessive pressure on the bladder, affecting urinary incontinence. Constipation can also lead to faecal incontinence as the pelvic floor muscles are weak, which can contribute to accidental bowel leakage.

During hypopressive training, the suction pressure in the abdominal cavity and the internal movement of the organs provides an internal massage that enhances blood flow encouraging more nutrients to enter the tissues, release toxins and stimulate the intestines to facilitate bowel movement. Hypopressive training, thus, can be a great tool in the treatment of constipation.[74,75]

Although not researched, there are other indirect benefits associated with the regular practice of hypopressives.

- Improved respiratory function
- Better sexual function
- Improved athletic performance
- Reduce waist perimeter
- Improve cardiovascular function and venous return
- Improve lymphatic system
- Create emotional balance and reduce stress levels
- Improve overall quality of life.

THE ABDOMINAL VACUUM

The hypopressive training system combines other techniques already existing and used by therapists. Risks are low; however, there are specific conditions in which performing the abdominal vacuum is not recommended for two main reasons:

1. Because we hold our breath for what could be considered an extended period (for more than five seconds), which has physiological effects on the body that can be negative or unknown in some conditions.

2. The inner traction of the organs and tissues in the abdominal and pelvic cavity could cause further harm to an existing condition.

WHEN NOT TO DO AN ABDOMINAL VACUUM:

- Pregnancy and immediate post-partum
- High blood pressure
- COPD (chronic obstructive pulmonary disease)
- Intestinal or gastric inflammations
- Cardiovascular or coronary problems
- Organ transplants
- Any medical contraindication to physical activity
- Recent surgical interventions
- Abdominal strangulated hernias
- Intra-uterine devices can move when performing abdominal vacuums
- Ehlers-Danlos Syndrome (a disorder that affects the connective tissues).

In any of these conditions, it is recommended to just perform DIAPHRAGMATIC BREATHING in the different poses, as described in the previous chapter.

HOW TO DO IT: STEP BY STEP

The following steps are a guide to try at home on your own, but to achieve optimal results, I recommend practising hypopressive exercises with a qualified instructor who can teach you the technique and make sure everything is done correctly.

Hypopressive training is performed by maintaining a sequence of postures that can be static or dynamic in a more advanced practice. Some of the basic poses have been described previously however, a greater repertoire of poses and actions can be added to the exercise sequence.

Each pose is maintained while performing THREE FULL DIAPHRAGMATIC BREATHING CYCLES AND ONE ABDOMINAL VACUUM. This is repeated three times per pose.

3 BREATHING CYCLES +1 ABDOMINAL VACUUM X3

And the exercise sequence is designed to commence with poses standing, then work your way down to the ground and finish lying down. A whole sequence lasts approximately 20 minutes.

TO PERFORM THE ABDOMINAL VACUUM:
STEP 1:

- Lie on your back with your legs bent and your hands on your ribs to feel your breathing movement.

- Do three diaphragmatic breathing cycles (inhale through your nose for the count of two, exhale through your mouth for the count of four). Remember to exhale with your mouth relaxed as if fogging a glass.

- On the third exhalation, slowly empty your lungs. Make sure you don't force the air out, bracing your abdominal muscles or bearing down. Compressing the core can be done as long as there is no bracing. This means you can feel your belly tightening, but not an outwards pressure.

• Visualise your core in this last exhale as if you were squeezing a toothpaste tube, flattening it upwards to push the air out of the body. Starting on your pelvic floor and continuing up pubic bone, belly button, diaphragm, lungs, throat and mouth.

• When you feel like you can't exhale any more, hold your breath for a few seconds. Then continue breathing.

• Repeat this cycle five more times, so you get used to the feeling of holding your breath with your lungs empty. Try to hold your breath for longer on each repetition.

STEP 2:

In this step, you will try to perform the vacuum.

• Perform the three breaths as described above.

• After the third exhalation, hold your breath by closing your mouth and pinching your nose so no air can get in.

• Now engage the vacuum by pretending to breathe in without actually letting any air in (think as if you were underwater and unable to inhale).

• Keep your abdominal wall relaxed and allow your ribs to expand in the same way as if you were taking a deep breath in (keep your shoulders and neck relaxed). Notice your abdominal wall automatically drawing in and up, experiencing a sucking feeling inside your stomach, perhaps accompanied by an inner stretch.

• Hold your breath for as long as possible (the longer, the better, but don't pass out!). Once you can't hold it anymore, gasp for air, slowly releasing the abdominal grip, letting your lungs fill with air in a controlled way. And continue breathing.

- Repeat this cycle ten times or as many times as you need. Remember that the key to feeling the abdominal vacuum is:

1) don't let any air into your airways, and

2) keep your abdominal wall relaxed (do not brace your abdominals as this will stop the vacuum from happening).

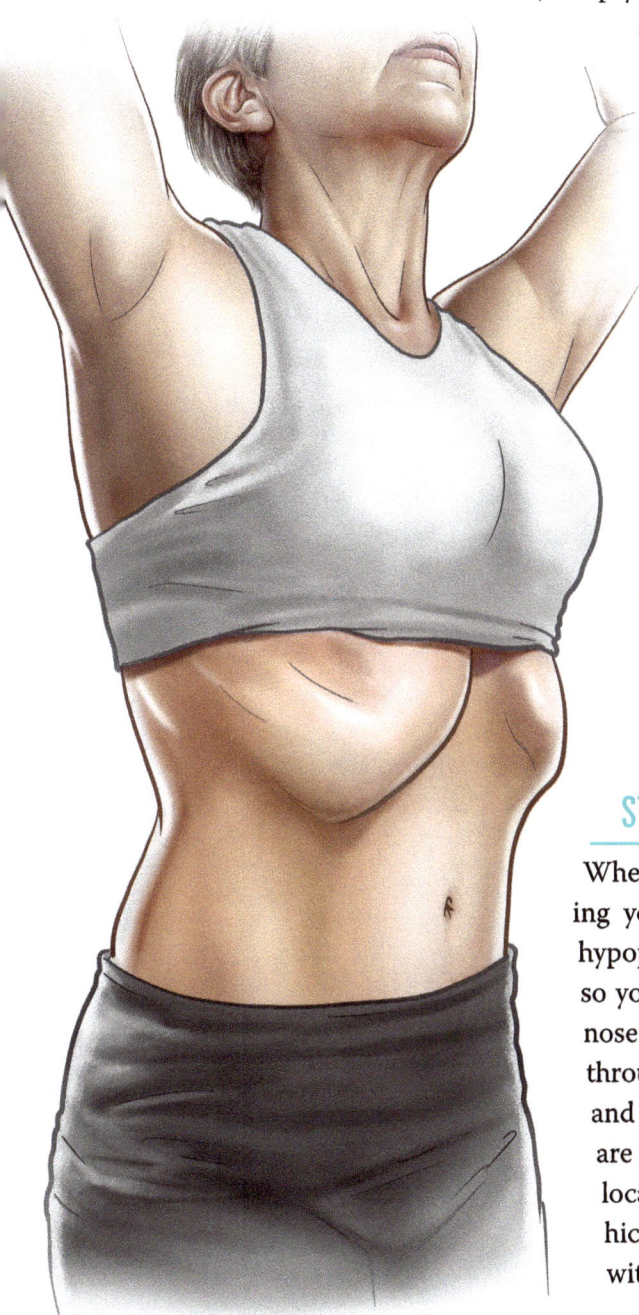

> **THIS IS WHAT AN ABDOMINAL VACUUM LOOKS LIKE.**

STEP 3:

When you have mastered Step 2, try it without pinching your nose. Ultimately, we want to incorporate hypopressive breathing into the exercise sequence, so you need to learn to do it without pinching your nose. To do this, you need to focus on NOT inhaling through your nose while pretending to breathe in and experiencing the rib expansion. For that you are required to close the airways through the glottis, located in your throat. It's similar to when you have hiccups, but this time is performed voluntarily and with control.

STEP 4:

Once you have mastered hypopressive breathing on the floor without having to pinch your nose you are ready to integrate it into the exercise sequence. You will do it by holding the poses described in the previous chapter.

- Hold the pose as you perform 3 to 4 breathing cycles (inhale through your nose for the count of 2, exhale through your mouth for the count of 4) and on the last exhalation, hold your breath to perform the abdominal vacuum.

- When you can't hold your breath any longer, gasp for air, but maintain the pose without moving.

- Repeat this sequence two more times in the same pose without resting.

- Once you have done three sets of vacuums, move on to the next pose and repeat the same sequence.

HOW DO I KNOW I'M DOING IT RIGHT?

Hypopressive breathing can be challenging to learn on your own. Even though it is a simple breathing modification, it is not an action we perform naturally.

Here are some signs that indicate whether you are doing hypopressive breathing correctly:

- While holding your breath, you can feel your ribs expanding out to the sides and your abdominal wall drawing in without you consciously pulling in.

- Your belly button moves in and up involuntarily, not because you are pulling it in.

- The space right underneath your ribs forms a slight hollow

- You experience a suction feeling around your neck and throat. This is different from experiencing an excess of tension in this area, which is undesirable.

- When you can no longer hold your breath, you feel the need to gasp for air. If you need to exhale, this means that at some point you have inhaled some air, and your lungs aren't empty, which prevents the vacuum from happening.

Things to pay attention to when performing hypopressive breathing:

- If you start feeling light-headed, it means that you are breathing too deeply and quickly, possibly even hyperventilating, causing you to feel dizzy. You need to slow down the rhythm of your breathing.

- Sometimes, people experience some neck pain during the exercises. This is common and means you are overactivating your neck and shoulders during the exercises. To prevent this, keep your face and neck muscles relaxed and focus on pulling your shoulders down and away from your ears while holding your breath.

- A common mistake during the deep exhale is to tighten the abdominal muscles to squeeze the last of the air out of your lungs. This can generate a pushing movement of the abdominal wall and is exactly what we need to avoid, so it is vital to focus on exhaling thoroughly while keeping the abdominal wall relaxed. To ensure your abdominal wall is relaxed, you can massage it while exhaling to check you are not tightening the muscles.

HYPOPRESSIVE TRAINING can be practised daily if desired; to experience its benefits, a minimum of two days a week for at least 12 weeks is required. And like any other training program, if you stop practising, some of the problems and conditions you were previously experiencing may come back after some time. It's a long-term commitment!

TRUST YOUR BODY

Awareness of the symbiotic relationship between your posture, breathing patterns, core and pelvic floor function can be very helpful, especially when dealing with dysfunction. It is likely that you have never paid attention to any of this until you experienced discomfort that drove you to seek help and information. And that is completely normal!

Bad posture and muscular imbalances affect every single task we do in our lives. Our bodies will always have muscular imbalances, just by the simple fact that we use mostly one arm and one leg for many things. But some of these imbalances, if we neglect them in the long term, our bodies start to adapt and create inefficient compensations that can lead to chronic pain and injuries.

OUR BODIES ARE SUPPOSED TO CARRY OUT THESE FUNCTIONS **AUTOMATICALLY,** SO WE SHOULDN'T HAVE TO THINK ABOUT HOW WE BREATHE, HOW WE STAND OR HOW OUR MUSCLES ENGAGE AND MODULATE TENSION AND PRESSURE DURING MOTION.

That's why hypervigilance or overthinking can sometimes bring more problems than benefits. It's very hard not to fall into this trap of insecurity and lack of trust in your own body when your symptoms constantly remind you that something is not right. But in most cases, overthinking leads to more insecurity and confusion. The complexity of the body doesn't allow us to control every single thing it does. Only when we relax and give our bodies a chance to do what they are supposed to do, we see the improvements. And that is what functionality truly means.

DON'T THINK — FEEL!

HYPOPRESSIVE TRAINING WITH PAULA

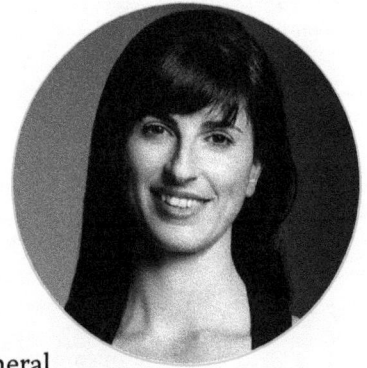

ACCESSIBLE CLASSES FOR EVERYONE

Paula provides Hypopressive training suitable for the general public, offering both in-person and online classes. Her training programs are carefully designed to accommodate all fitness levels and health objectives. Whether your goal is post-birth recovery, improvement of posture, injury management, or performance development, Paula tailors her methods to address each individual's unique needs.

PROFESSIONAL DEVELOPMENT OPPORTUNITIES

As a founding member of the International Hypopressive Council, Paula also delivers specialised courses for fitness and health professionals interested in incorporating the Hypopressive Method into their practice. Participants in these courses include regular and pelvic floor physiotherapists, osteopaths, chiropractors, exercise physiologists, midwives, doulas, Pilates and Yoga instructors, bodybuilding coaches, personal trainers, and sports coaches.

CONTACT AND SOCIAL MEDIA

To connect with Paula:-

🌐 paulacampanero.com

✉️ paula@paulacampanero.com

For updates and insights, follow her on:-

f Core Tone Fitness

📷 @coretonehypopressivesaustralia

To learn about Hypopressives in the world, visit the International Hypopressive Council Website hypopressivesinternational.com

REFERENCES

1. Australian Institute of Health and Welfare. Incontinence in Australia. Canberra; 2013.

2. Hannestad YS, Rortveit G, Hunskaar S. Help-seeking and associated factors in female urinary incontinence. The Norwegian EPINCONT Study. Ep.... Scand J Prim Health Care [Internet]. [cited 2023 Mar 14]; Available from: https://pubmed.ncbi.nlm.nih.gov/12184708/

3. Research update. Pelvic organ prolapse physiotherapy. Australian and New Zealand Continence Journal. 2000 Jun;14(2):50–5.

4. Bø K, Sundgot Borgen J. Prevalence of stress and urge urinary incontinence in elite athletes and controls [Internet]. Vol. 33, Med. Sci. Sports Exerc. 2001. Available from: http://journals.lww.com/acsm-msse

5. Bush HM, Pagorek S, Kuperstein J, Guo J, Ballert KN, Crofford LJ. The Association of Chronic Back Pain and Stress Urinary Incontinence: A Cross-Sectional Study.

6. Barton A, Serrao C, Thompson J, Briffa K. Transabdominal ultrasound to assess pelvic floor muscle performance during abdominal curl in exercising women. Int Urogynecol J [Internet]. 2015 Dec 1 [cited 2023 Mar 17];26(12):1789–95. Available from: https://link.springer.com/article/10.1007/s00192-015-2791-9

7. Lederman E. The Myth of Core Stability. [cited 2023 Mar 17]; Available from: www.cpdo.net

8. Body Weight and Low Back Pain: A Systematic Literature Revie... : Spine [Internet]. [cited 2023 Mar 17]. Available from: https://journals.lww.com/spinejournal/Abstract/2000/01150/Body_Weight_and_Low_Back_Pain__A_Systematic.15.aspx

9. White SG, McNair PJ. Abdominal and erector spinae muscle activity during gait: The use of cluster analysis to identify patterns of activity. Clinical Biomechanics [Internet]. 2002 Mar 1 [cited 2023 Mar 20];17(3):177–84. Available from: http://www.clinbiomech.com/article/S0268003302000074/fulltext

10. Hubley-Kozey CL, Vezina MJ. Muscle activation during exercises to improve trunk stability in men with low back pain. Arch Phys Med Rehabil. 2002 Aug 1;83(8):1100–8.

11. Souza GM, Baker LL, Powers CM. Electromyographic activity of selected trunk muscles during dynamic spine stabilization exercises. Arch Phys Med Rehabil [Internet]. 2001 Nov 1 [cited 2023 Mar 20];82(11):1551–7. Available from: http://www.archives-pmr.org/article/S0003999301440482/fulltext

12. De Keulenaer BL, De Waele JJ, Powell B, Malbrain MLNG. What is normal intra-abdominal pressure and how is it affected by positioning, body mass and positive end-expiratory pressure? Vol. 35, Intensive Care Medicine. 2009. p. 969–76.

13. Hamad NM, Shaw JM, Nygaard IE, Coleman TJ, Hsu Y, Egger M, et al. More complicated than it looks: The vagaries of calculating intra-abdominal pressure. J Strength Cond Res [Internet]. 2013 [cited 2023 Mar 21];27(11):3204–15. Available from: https://journals.lww.com/nsca-jscr/Fulltext/2013/11000/More_Complicated_Than_it_Looks__The_Vagaries_of.35.aspx

14. Egger MJ, Hamad NM, Hitchcock RW, Coleman TJ, Shaw JM, Hsu Y, et al. Reproducibility of intra-abdominal pressure measured during physical activities via a wireless vaginal transducer. Female Pelvic Med Reconstr Surg. 2015 May 9;21(3):164–9.

15. Caix M, Outrequin G, Descottes B, Kalfon M, Pouget X. The muscles of the abdominal wall: a new functional approach with anatomoclinical deductions. Vol. 6, Anat Clin. Springer-Verlag; 1984.

16. Hwang YI, Kim KS. Effects of pelvic tilt angles and forced vital capacity in healthy individuals. J Phys Ther Sci [Internet]. 2018 [cited 2023 Mar 27];30(1):82. Available from: /pmc/articles/PMC5788781/

17. Kannan P, Winser S, Goonetilleke R, Cheing G. Ankle positions potentially facilitating greater maximal contraction of pelvic floor muscles: a systematic review and meta-analysis. https://doi.org/101080/0963828820181468934 [Internet]. 2018 Oct 9 [cited 2023 Mar 27];41(21):2483–91. Available from: https://www.tandfonline.com/doi/abs/10.1080/09638288.2018.1468934

18. Junginger B, Baessler K, Sapsford R, Hodges PW. Effect of abdominal and pelvic floor tasks on muscle activity, abdominal pressure and bladder neck. Int Urogynecol J [Internet]. 2010 Sep 3 [cited 2023 Mar 27];21(1):69–77. Available from: https://link.springer.com/article/10.1007/s00192-009-0981-z

19. Neumann P, Gill V. Pelvic floor and abdominal muscle interaction: EMG activity and intra-abdominal pressure. Int Urogynecol J [Internet]. 2002 Mar 18 [cited 2023 Mar 27];13(2):125–32. Available from: https://link.springer.com/article/10.1007/s001920200027

20. Sapsford R. Rehabilitation of pelvic floor muscles utilizing trunk stabilization. Man Ther. 2004 Feb 1;9(1):3–12.

21. Da Roza T, De Araujo MP, Viana R, Viana S, Jorge RN, Bø K, et al. Pelvic floor muscle training to improve urinary incontinence in young, nulliparous sport students: A pilot study. Int Urogynecol J [Internet]. 2012 May 3 [cited 2023 Mar 28];23(8):1069–73. Available from: https://link.springer.com/article/10.1007/s00192-012-1759-2

22. de Mattos Lourenco TR, Matsuoka PK, Baracat EC, Haddad JM. Urinary incontinence in female athletes: a systematic review. Int Urogynecol J [Internet]. 2018 Dec 1 [cited 2023 Mar 28];29(12):1757–63. Available from: https://link.springer.com/article/10.1007/s00192-018-3629-z

23. Bø K, Bratland-Sanda S, Sundgot-Borgen J. Urinary incontinence among group fitness instructors including yoga and pilates teachers. Neurourol Urodyn [Internet]. 2011 Mar 1 [cited 2023 Mar 28];30(3):370–3. Available from: https://onlinelibrary.wiley.com/doi/full/10.1002/nau.21006

24. Nygaard I, DeLancey JO, Arnsdorf L, Murphy E. Exercise and incontinence. Obstetrics and gynecology. 1990 May;75(5):848–51.

25. Jácome C, Oliveira D, Marques A, Sá-Couto P. Prevalence and impact of urinary incontinence among female athletes. International Journal of Gynecology & Obstetrics [Internet]. 2011 Jul 1 [cited 2023 Mar 28];114(1):60–3. Available from: https://onlinelibrary.wiley.com/doi/full/10.1016/j.ijgo.2011.02.004

26. Nygaard IE. Does prolonged high-impact activity contribute to later urinary incontinence? A retrospective cohort study of female olympians. Obstetrics & Gynecology. 1997 Nov 1;90(5):718–22.

27. Eliasson K, Edner A, Mattsson E. Urinary incontinence in very young and mostly nulliparous women with a history of regular organised high-impact trampoline training: Occurrence and risk factors. Int Urogynecol J [Internet]. 2008 Jan 26 [cited 2023 Mar 28];19(5):687–96. Available from: https://link.springer.com/article/10.1007/s00192-007-0508-4

28. Thompson JA, O'Sullivan PB, Briffa NK, Neumann P. Comparison of transperineal and transabdominal ultrasound in the assessment of voluntary pelvic floor muscle contractions and functional manoeuvres in continent and incontinent women. Int Urogynecol J [Internet]. 2007 Oct 17 [cited 2023 Mar 28];18(7):779–86. Available from: https://link.springer.com/article/10.1007/s00192-006-0225-4

29. Simpson S, Deeble M, Thompson J, Andrews A, Briffa K. Should women with incontinence and prolapse do abdominal curls? Int Urogynecol J [Internet]. 2016 Oct 1 [cited 2023 Mar 28];27(10):1507–12. Available from: https://link.springer.com/article/10.1007/s00192-016-3005-9

30. Bø K, Stien R. Needle emg registration of striated urethral wall and pelvic floor muscle activity patterns during cough, valsalva, abdominal, hip adductor, and gluteal muscle contractions in nulliparous healthy females. Neurourol Urodyn [Internet]. 1994 Jan 1 [cited 2023 Mar 28];13(1):35–41. Available from: https://onlinelibrary.wiley.com/doi/full/10.1002/nau.1930130106

31. Neumann P, Gill V. Pelvic floor and abdominal muscle interaction: EMG activity and intra-abdominal pressure. Int Urogynecol J [Internet]. 2002 Mar 18 [cited 2023 Mar 28];13(2):125–32. Available from: https://link.springer.com/article/10.1007/s001920200027

32. Pelvic Floor Disorders: The Role of Fascia and Ligaments : Clinical Obstetrics and Gynecology [Internet]. [cited 2023 Apr 3]. Available from: https://journals.lww.com/clinicalobgyn/Citation/1993/12000/Pelvic_Floor_Disorders__The_Role_of_Fascia_and.17.aspx

33. Lammers K, Lince SL, Spath MA, VanKempen LCLT, Hendriks JCM, Vierhout ME, et al. Pelvic organ prolapse and collagen-associated disorders. Int Urogynecol J [Internet]. 2012 Aug 3 [cited 2023 Apr 3];23(3):313–9. Available from: https://link.springer.com/article/10.1007/s00192-011-1532-y

34. Iglesia CB, Sokol AI, Sokol ER, Kudish BI, Gutman RE, Peterson JL, et al. Vaginal Mesh for Prolapse. Obstetrics & Gynecology. 2010 Aug;116(2):293–303.

35. Ismail SI, Bain C, Hagen S. Oestrogens for treatment or prevention of pelvic organ prolapse in postmenopausal women. Cochrane Database of Systematic Reviews [Internet]. 2010 Sep 8 [cited 2023 Apr 3];(9). Available from: https://www.cochranelibrary.com/cdsr/doi/10.1002/14651858.CD007063.pub2/full

36. Gong R, Xia Z. Collagen changes in pelvic support tissues in women with pelvic organ prolapse. European Journal of Obstetrics and Gynecology and Reproductive Biology [Internet]. 2019 Mar 1 [cited 2023 Apr 3];234:185–9. Available from: http://www.ejog.org/article/S0301211519300399/fulltext

37. Khatri M, Naughton RJ, Clifford T, Harper LD, Corr L. The effects of collagen peptide supplementation on body composition, collagen synthesis, and recovery from joint injury and exercise: a systematic review. Amino Acids [Internet]. 2021 Oct 1 [cited 2023 Apr 3];53(10):1493–506. Available from: https://link.springer.com/article/10.1007/s00726-021-03072-x

38. Miller BF, Hansen M, Olesen JL, Schwarz P, Babraj JA, Smith K, et al. Tendon collagen synthesis at rest and after exercise in women. J Appl Physiol. 2007 Feb;102(2):541–6.

39. Langberg H, Rosendal L, Kjær M. Training-induced changes in peritendinous type I collagen turnover determined by microdialysis in humans. J Physiol. 2001 Jul;534(1):297–302.

40. Shaw G, Lee-Barthel A, Ross MLR, Wang B, Baar K. Vitamin C–enriched gelatin supplementation before intermittent activity augments collagen synthesis,. Am J Clin Nutr. 2017 Jan 1;105(1):136–43.

41. Diastasis Rectus Abdominis and Lumbo-Pelvic Pain and Dysfunc... : Journal of Women's & Pelvic Health Physical Therapy [Internet]. [cited 2023 Apr 5]. Available from: https://journals.lww.com/jwhpt/Abstract/2009/33020/Diastasis_Rectus_Abdominis_and_Lumbo_Pelvic_Pain.3.aspx

42. Fei H, Liu Y, Li M, He J, Liu L, Li J, et al. The relationship of severity in diastasis recti abdominis and pelvic floor dysfunction: a retrospective cohort study. BMC Womens Health [Internet]. 2021 Dec 1 [cited 2023 Apr 5];21(1):1–8. Available from: https://bmcwomenshealth.biomedcentral.com/articles/10.1186/s12905-021-01194-8

43. Bø K, Hilde G, Tennfjord MK, Sperstad JB, Engh ME. Pelvic floor muscle function, pelvic floor dysfunction and diastasis recti abdominis: Prospective cohort study. Neurourol Urodyn [Internet]. 2017 Mar 1 [cited 2023 Apr 11];36(3):716–21. Available from: https://onlinelibrary.wiley.com/doi/full/10.1002/nau.23005

44. Co-activation of the abdominal and pelvic floor muscles during voluntary exercises - Sapsford - 2001 - Neurourology and Urodynamics - Wiley Online Library [Internet]. [cited 2023 Apr 11]. Available from: https://onlinelibrary.wiley.com/doi/10.1002/1520-6777(2001)20:1%3C31::AID-NAU5%3E3.0.CO;2-P

45. Cavalli M, Aiolfi A, Bruni PG, Manfredini L, Lombardo F, Bonfanti MT, et al. Prevalence and risk factors for diastasis recti abdominis: a review and proposal of a new anatomical variation. Hernia [Internet]. 2021 Aug 1 [cited 2023 Apr 11];25(4):883–90. Available from: https://link.springer.com/article/10.1007/s10029-021-02468-8

46. Benjamin DR, van de Water ATM, Peiris CL. Effects of exercise on diastasis of the rectus abdominis muscle in the antenatal and postnatal periods: A systematic review. Physiotherapy (United Kingdom) [Internet]. 2014 Mar 1 [cited 2023 Apr 11];100(1):1–8. Available from: http://www.physiotherapyjournal.com/article/S0031940613000837/fulltext

47. Lee D, Hodges PW. Behavior of the linea alba during a curl-up task in diastasis rectus abdominis: An observational study. Journal of Orthopaedic and Sports Physical Therapy [Internet]. 2016 Jul 1 [cited 2023 Apr 11];46(7):580–9. Available from: https://www.jospt.org/doi/10.2519/jospt.2016.6536

48. Mota P, Pascoal AG, Carita AI, Kari B. The immediate effects on inter-rectus distance of abdominal crunch and drawing-in exercises during pregnancy and the postpartum period. Journal of Orthopaedic and Sports Physical Therapy [Internet]. 2015 Oct 1 [cited 2023 Apr 11];45(10):781–8. Available from: https://www.jospt.org/doi/10.2519/jospt.2015.5459

49. Kingsnorth A, LeBlanc K. Hernias: inguinal and incisional. The Lancet [Internet]. 2003 Nov 8 [cited 2023 Apr 11];362(9395):1561–71. Available from: http://www.thelancet.com/article/S0140673603147460/fulltext

50. Sports Hernia: Diagnosis and Therapeutic Approach : JAAOS - Journal of the American Academy of Orthopaedic Surgeons [Internet]. [cited 2023 Apr 11]. Available from: https://journals.lww.com/jaaos/Abstract/2007/08000/Sports_Hernia__Diagnosis_and_Therapeutic_Approach.7.aspx

51. Schroeder GD, Guyre CA, Vaccaro AR. The epidemiology and pathophysiology of lumbar disc herniations. Semin Spine Surg. 2016 Mar 1;28(1):2–7.

52. Marshall LW, McGill SM. The role of axial torque in disc herniation. Clinical Biomechanics [Internet]. 2010 Jan 1 [cited 2023 Apr 12];25(1):6–9. Available from: http://www.clinbiomech.com/article/S0268003309002162/fulltext

53. Fjeld OR, Grøvle L, Helgeland J, Småstuen MC, Solberg TK, Zwart JA, et al. Complications, reoperations, readmissions, and length of hospital stay in 34 639 surgical cases of lumbar disc herniation. Bone Joint J. 2019 Apr 1;101-B(4):470–7.

54.   Santa Mina D, Au D, Alibhai SMH, Jamnicky L, Faghani N, Hilton WJ, et al. A pilot randomized trial of conventional versus advanced pelvic floor exercises to treat urinary incontinence after radical prostatectomy: a study protocol. BMC Urol [Internet]. 2015 Sep 16 [cited 2023 Apr 12];15(1):94–94. Available from: https://europepmc.org/articles/PMC4574075

55.   Ma X, Yue ZQ, Gong ZQ, Zhang H, Duan NY, Shi YT, et al. The Effect of Diaphragmatic Breathing on Attention, Negative Affect and Stress in Healthy Adults. Front Psychol. 2017 Jun 6;8.

56.   Effects of diafragamatic aspiration on physical and blood parametres of professional mountain bikers | Request PDF [Internet]. [cited 2023 Apr 14]. Available from: https://www.researchgate.net/publication/289576125_Effects_of_diafragamatic_aspiration_on_physical_and_blood_parametres_of_professional_mountain_bikers

57.   (PDF) Can an eight-week program based on the hypopressive technique produce changes in pelvic floor function and body composition in female rugby players? [Internet]. [cited 2023 Apr 14]. Available from: https://www.researchgate.net/publication/296195440_Can_an_eight-week_program_based_on_the_hypopressive_technique_produce_changes_in_pelvic_floor_function_and_body_composition_in_female_rugby_players

58.   Resende APM, Stüpp L, Bernardes BT, Oliveira E, Castro RA, Girão MJBC, et al. Can hypopressive exercises provide additional benefits to pelvic floor muscle training in women with pelvic organ prolapse? Neurourol Urodyn [Internet]. 2012 Jan 1 [cited 2023 Apr 14];31(1):121–5. Available from: https://onlinelibrary.wiley.com/doi/full/10.1002/nau.21149

59.   Sutter Latorre GF, Regina Seleme M, Magalhães Resenda AP, Stüpp L, Berghmans B. Hypopressive Gymnastics: Evidences for an Alternative Training for Women with Local Proprioceptive Deficit of the Pelvic Floor Muscles. Fisioterapia Brasil. 2011 Nov;12(6):463–6.

60.   Navarro-Brazález B, Prieto-Gómez V, Prieto-Merino D, Sánchez-Sánchez B, McLean L, Torres-Lacomba M. Effectiveness of Hypopressive Exercises in Women with Pelvic Floor Dysfunction: A Randomised Controlled Trial. J Clin Med. 2020 Apr 17;9(4):1149.

61.   Mateus-Vasconcelos ECL, Ribeiro AM, Antônio FI, Brito LG de O, Ferreira CHJ. Physiotherapy methods to facilitate pelvic floor muscle contraction: A systematic review. Physiother Theory Pract. 2018 Jun 3;34(6):420–32.

62.   Molina-Torres G, Moreno-Muñoz M, Rebullido TR, Castellote-Caballero Y, Bergamin M, Gobbo S, et al. The effects of an 8-week hypopressive exercise training program on urinary incontinence and pelvic floor muscle activation: A randomized controlled trial. Neurourol Urodyn [Internet]. 2023 Feb 1 [cited 2023 Apr 17];42(2):500–9. Available from: https://onlinelibrary.wiley.com/doi/full/10.1002/nau.25110

63.   Omkar SN, Vishwas S. Yoga techniques as a means of core stability training. J Bodyw Mov Ther [Internet]. 2009 Jan 1 [cited 2023 Apr 17];13(1):98–103. Available from: http://www.bodyworkmovementtherapies.com/article/S1360859207001106/fulltext

64.   Da Cuña-Carrera I, Alonso-calvete A, Soto-gonzález M, Lantarón-caeiro EM. How Do the Abdominal Muscles Change during Hypopressive Exercise? Medicina 2021, Vol 57, Page 702 [Internet]. 2021 Jul 9 [cited 2023 Apr 17];57(7):702. Available from: https://www.mdpi.com/1648-9144/57/7/702/htm

65.   Ithamar L, de Moura Filho AG, Benedetti Rodrigues MA, Duque Cortez KC, Machado VG, de Paiva Lima CRO, et al. Abdominal and pelvic floor electromyographic analysis during abdominal hypopressive gymnastics. J Bodyw Mov Ther [Internet]. 2018 Jan 1 [cited 2023 Apr 17];22(1):159–65. Available from: http://www.bodyworkmovementtherapies.com/article/S1360859217301353/fulltext

66. Au D, Matthew AG, Alibhai SMH, Jones JM, Fleshner NE, Finelli A, et al. Pfilates and Hypopressives for the Treatment of Urinary Incontinence After Radical Prostatectomy: Results of a Feasibility Randomized Controlled Trial. PM&R [Internet]. 2020 Jan 1 [cited 2023 Apr 17];12(1):55–63. Available from: https://onlinelibrary.wiley.com/doi/full/10.1002/pmrj.12157

67. Santa Mina D, Au D, Alibhai SMH, Jamnicky L, Faghani N, Hilton WJ, et al. A pilot randomized trial of conventional versus advanced pelvic floor exercises to treat urinary incontinence after radical prostatectomy: A study protocol. BMC Urol [Internet]. 2015 Sep 16 [cited 2023 Apr 17];15(1):1–10. Available from: https://bmcurol.biomedcentral.com/articles/10.1186/s12894-015-0088-4

68. Rial Rebullido T, Chulvi Medrano I. A case study of hypopressive exercise adapted for urinary incontinence following radical prostatectomy surgery. Fisioterapia. 2018;40(20).

69. Ramírez-Jiménez M, Alburquerque-Sendín F, Garrido-Castro JL, Rodrigues-de-Souza D. Effects of hypopressive exercises on post-partum abdominal diastasis, trunk circumference, and mechanical properties of abdominopelvic tissues: a case series. Physiother Theory Pract. 2023 Jan;39(1):49–60.

70. Cuña Carrera I da, González González Y, Lantarón Caeiro EM, Soto González M. Efectos de diferentes ejercicios abdominales en la distancia interrectos. Revista Internacional de Deportes Colectivos, ISSN-e 1989-841X, No 35, 2018, págs 43-52 [Internet]. 2018 [cited 2023 Apr 17];(35):43–52. Available from: https://dialnet.unirioja.es/servlet/articulo?codigo=6749919&info=resumen&idioma=ENG

71. Gómez FR, Senín-Camargo FJ, Cancela-Cores Á, Patiño-Núñez S, Carballo-Costa L. C0083 Effect of a hipopressive abdominal exercise program on inter-rectus abdominis muscles distance in postpartum. In: Abstracts. BMJ Publishing Group Ltd and British Association of Sport and Exercise Medicine; 2018. p. A21.2-A21.

72. Bellido-Fernández L, Jiménez-Rejano JJ, Chillón-Martínez R, Gómez-Benítez MA, De-La-Casa-Almeida M, Rebollo-Salas M. Effectiveness of Massage Therapy and Abdominal Hypopressive Gymnastics in Nonspecific Chronic Low Back Pain: A Randomized Controlled Pilot Study. Evid Based Complement Alternat Med [Internet]. 2018 [cited 2023 Apr 17];2018. Available from: /pmc/articles/PMC5842706/

73. Moreno-Muñoz MDM, Hita-Contreras F, Estudillo-Martínez MD, Aibar-Almazán A, Castellote-Caballero Y, Bergamin M, et al. The Effects of Abdominal Hypopressive Training on Postural Control and Deep Trunk Muscle Activation: A Randomized Controlled Trial. Int J Environ Res Public Health [Internet]. 2021 Mar 1 [cited 2023 Apr 17];18(5):1–13. Available from: /pmc/articles/PMC7967465/

74. Fernandez et al. The effects of gymnastics abdominal hypopressives in women with constipation. Cinergis. 2014;15(3):148–51.

75. Mishra SP, Singh RH. EFFECT OF CERTAIN YOGIC ASANAS ON THE PELVIC CONGESTION AND IT'S ANATOMY. Anc Sci Life [Internet]. 1984 [cited 2023 Apr 17];4(2):127. Available from: /pmc/articles/PMC3331493/?report=abstract

OTHER REFERENCES:

1. Busquet L, Las cadenas musculares: Tronco y columna cervical (The muscle chains trunk and spine). 2004 Paidotribo.

2. Calais-Germain B. El perine femenino y el parto. Elementos de anatomia y bases de ejercicios. 12th ed. Barcelona: La Liebre de Marzo 2016.

3. Houser E.E, Riley Hahn S. A woman's guide to pelvic health. Baltimore: The John's Hopkins University Press; 2012.

4. Lee D. The pelvic girdle – An integration of clinical expertise and research. 4th ed. Churcill Livingstone; 2011.

5. Myers T. Anatomy trains: Myofascial meridians for manual and movement therapists. 3rd ed. Churchill Livingstone; 2014.

6. O' Dwyer M. Hold it mama: The pelvic floor and core handbook for pregnancy, birth and beyond. Australia. Red Sok; 2012.

7. Riat T, Pinsach P. Hypopressive techniques. Vigo (Spain). Editorial Cardenoso; 2015.

8. Rial T, Pinsach P. Practical manual of hypopressives Level 1. Vigo (Spain). Editorial Cardenoso; 2015.

ONLINE REFERENCES:

- Gibson J. Chronic prostatitis/ Chronic pelvic pain syndrome [Internet]. San Francisco. 2012.
  Available from: http://malepelvicfloor.com/cpps.html

- Gibson J. Sexual dysfunction and genital pain [Internet]. San Francisco. 2012.
  Available from: http://malepelvicfloor.com/sd.html

- Vopni K – Bellies Inc. Diastasis recti and the pelvic floor connection [Internet]. Bump 2 Baby Ontario. Klusster; March 2019. Available from: https://www.klusster.com/klussters/bump-2-baby-ontario/publications/diastas-is-recti-and-the-pelvic-floor-connection-1448-5981

- Burrell J. Burrell Education: What actually improves diastasis [Internet]. Facebook. 1 July 2019.
  Available from: https://www.facebook.com/burrelleducation/videos/498711660697697/

- Burrell J. Burrell Education: Do you know how to test for a functional diastasis? [Internet]. Facebook 18 Feb 2019. Available from: https://www.facebook.com/burrelleducation/videos/776863502692435/

www.ingramcontent.com/pod-product-compliance
Lightning Source LLC
Chambersburg PA
CBHW051617030426

42334CB00030B/3231